Infinite Resignation:

The Art of an Infant Heart Transplant

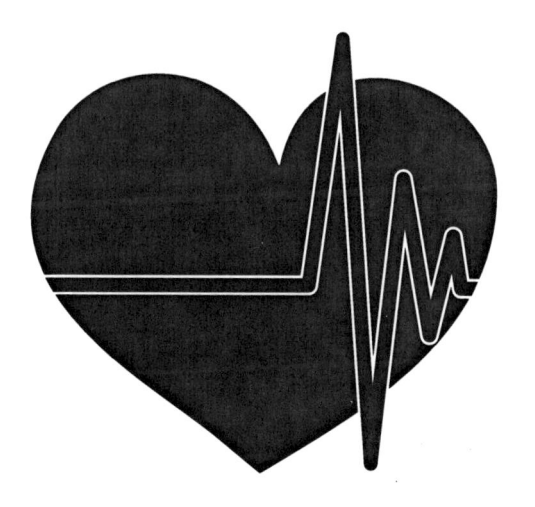

Ernest Kroeker

Copyright © 2013 by Ernest Kroeker
First Edition – November 2013

ISBN
978-1-4602-2510-3 (Hardcover)
978-1-4602-2511-0 (Paperback)
978-1-4602-2512-7 (eBook)

All rights reserved.

No part of this publication may be reproduced in any form, or by any means, electronic or mechanical, including photocopying, recording, or any information browsing, storage, or retrieval system, without permission in writing from the publisher.

Produced by:

FriesenPress
Suite 300 – 852 Fort Street
Victoria, BC, Canada V8W 1H8

www.friesenpress.com

Distributed to the trade by The Ingram Book Company

For Mark and for the 16 month old girl who died on September 28, 1989 somewhere near Los Angeles, CA. Her heart still beats in Mark's chest.

Introduction
All my dreams

It was one of those magical moments in life that remains embedded in my mind as fresh as if it just happened yesterday. A group of friends were sitting together in an old farmhouse on the edge of a quaint village. It was early in the evening and we had just eaten a lovely dinner with enough wine that everyone was uninhibited but not silly. Suddenly there was a dramatic pause in all the conversations around the room; everyone stopped talking at the same time with the exception of one young woman who was engrossed in a conversation with a particular young man. "So what are your dreams for your life?" she asked as she turned and noticed that the room had gone quiet and everyone was now looking at her. It was as if she was addressing the whole room and after we overcame our amusement we all decided that it was a great question and that we should go around the room and provide our own answers.

Most of the people present were young university students so the answers were quite interesting.

I had some time to consider what I was going to say as I happened to be one of the last in line to respond. At first I was a little shaken by the question. What would I say? Should I admit to my secret ambition to sing at the *Met*?

Should I reveal all and tell them about my crazy notion to one day represent my country at an international dressage competition? In the end I decided to keep it simple and straightforward. When my turn came I said that what I wanted most of all in life was a house full of children and a barn full of horses.

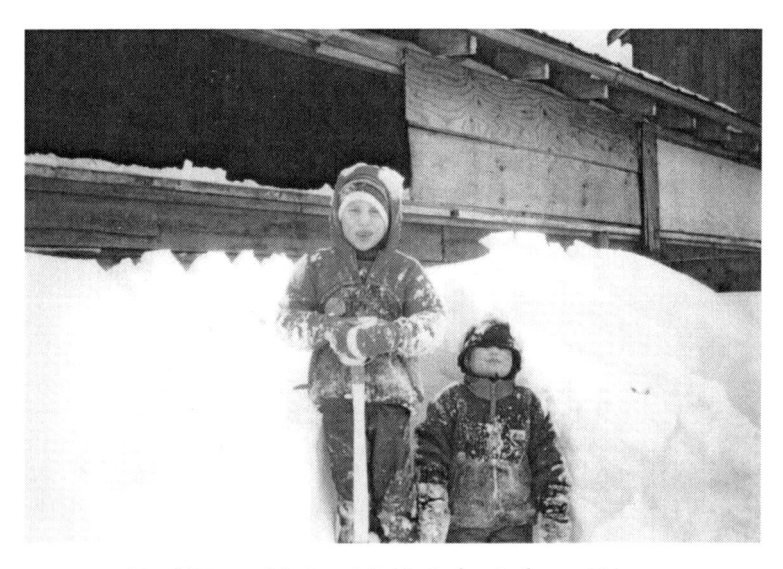

My children – Mark and Robin in front of our old barn

Twelve years later I was sitting in the lobby of the university hospital in Saskatoon, Saskatchewan. It was late afternoon and people were coming and going. Many hospital personnel were arriving for the evening shift and visitors were coming in to see sick friends and family. For me it was as if the whole place was full of white noise because I was in shock. I had just had the worst day of my life. My wife and I had spent most of the day in the paediatric cardiology department where we had been informed that our unborn child, the object of our dreams would die of a fatal heart condition shortly after birth. A great ball of sickening dread was sitting at the very center of my being. The team of cardiologists had given us little hope that this could end well.

I had made very little progress in terms of achieving the objects of my dreams in the twelve years since that memorable night in the farmhouse. My chances of ever singing at the *Met* had been essentially ruined by doing Bob Dylan impersonations for several years. I had however sung at *La Scala* – nothing too formal or official. While visiting Milan with a friend we had tried to tour this prestigious institution but had found the whole building locked up tight. We were having drinks at a sidewalk cafe to deal with our disappointment when we noticed two maintenance workers leave the building via a side door. They were obviously taking a break and left the door ajar so that they could return. I saw this as my chance at the big time. I slipped through the door and made a brief tour of the building. I discovered a doorway to the main stage and had just started singing when the workers returned. They apparently alerted security and I was not able to finish one of my better renditions of *Un'ombra di Pace* before I was ushered out of the building. I insisted on leaving through the front door.

My accomplishments in the equestrian world had not been stellar either. I had spent some time at a reputable riding academy in Europe and had actually sat on a horse while it performed *piaffe* and passage, but riding an entire Grand Prix dressage test from start to finish still remains near the top of my list of things to do.

To my surprise however, becoming the proud owner of a barn full of horses and the father of a house full of children - these supposedly simple and straightforward dreams - had proven even more difficult to achieve than the even wilder fantasies. I had spent my time at several different universities accumulating various degrees of success. I had eventually finished writing a PhD thesis and had convinced my committee they might be willing to give me this degree. In anticipation of this event I had taken up my first real job at the University of Saskatchewan as a research associate. Because this was not a permanent position, I had rented a small house on a farmyard. Included in the deal was the use of an even smaller barn. I would at least have the necessary infrastructure for my dreams in place. Neither the house nor the barn was very large so they would not be that hard to fill. I had also managed to convince a beautiful, very intelligent young woman that I might make a good mate and her pregnancy was living proof that if things are meant to be, they work out even the very first time you try. Or do they? Just six months into the pregnancy the dream had come crashing down in one single horrible day. Our child was going to die and I realized that I had never before felt the real devastation or absolute dread that I did that day.

Chapter 1
Birth or Death?

Were we lead all that way for
Birth or death? There was a Birth, certainly,
We had evidence and no doubt. I had seen birth and death,
But had thought they were different; this Birth was
Hard and bitter agony for us, like Death, our death.

T.S. Eliot, *Journey of the Magi*

I had seen many births and also some death in preparation for the birth of our first child. I grew up on a large farm where our family kept a variety of different animals: chickens, horses, pigs, but mostly cows which produced marketable products most efficiently. Every summer we would allow several bantam hens to sit on large nests of eggs and sometimes we were lucky enough to see the eggs hatch. It was magical to watch the chicks emerge all wet and sticky and then quickly dry off and turn into fluffy balls of pale yellow feathers. The cows gave birth regularly so that they would keep producing milk and cream to sell. The birth of a calf was always cause for great excitement and as soon as my siblings and I would hear of such an event, we would rush out to the barn, often still in our pyjamas, to see the new calf tottering around making its first awkward attempts at nursing.

As a child I was always frustrated that birth almost always occurred at night or while I was at school so I never actually got to see it. When I was a teenager however I started to witness calf births quite regularly and quickly learned to assist in the process when necessary. If a cow was straining too long and labour was not progressing I would put on long plastic gloves and reach in through her open cervix and check that I could find the two front feet and nose in the birth canal. If this was not the case something had to be done quickly; the closest vet was hours away so I learned to reach in and reposition the calf if possible.

My father actually preferred to let me do this because my hands and arms were much smaller than his were. Sometimes it was a simple task of finding a missing front foot and grasping the bottom of the leg and, trying to cover the little hoof to stop it from scraping against the uterus of the mother, carefully pulling it forward. If the head was bent back the task was usually much more difficult. You had to try to get your fingers into the nostrils of the calf and pull the head around – not that easy especially if you happened to have your arm in there during a contraction. I quickly learned that the uterus is one mother of a powerful muscle capable of seizing off the circulation in your arm and during such a contraction you better get your arms out of there as quickly as possible. Breach position with the hind legs and hips coming first was the most difficult and usually required two strong individuals. I would tie thin soft cotton ropes to each back ankle and then my father would help to pull. On rare occasions we would be unsuccessful and the vet would arrive too late and the calf or the cow or both would die.

I had certainly witnessed enough birth and even death early in life so attending prenatal classes was a bit anticlimactic for me – that is until they showed the movie at the last session. Until then there was a lot of gentle talk about breathing and flowers opening and how wonderful the birth process is. It was only at the very end, after the movie, that the discussion shifted to the pros and cons of pain management and then trying to answer frantic questions like, "Why can't I just have a C-section?" Still, I got some very useful information and printed material about the role of the labour coach and a list of things to have packed and ready to go at a moment's notice.

In our case, the journey from conception to delivery had been very long and difficult, for our son had been diagnosed *in utero* with a congenital heart defect which would cause certain death in a matter of hours or days following his birth. The pregnancy had been declared high risk and we had travelled from our home in Saskatoon, Canada to southern California where we were hoping we might be able to get medical treatment for his condition after he was born. Like the Magi we had had a particularly difficult journey and we were not at all certain if the outcome would be a birth or a death.

Shortly before 6 pm on September 20th, 1989, my wife Nicole, her mother Janet, who had come down to act as back-up coach, and I were sitting at the kitchen table in a small apartment in Redlands, CA - a completely foreign land. We had had dinner and were playing cards to pass the time when Nicole started to feel a lot of activity in her abdomen. At 6:19 the contractions started to become quite regular so I began to keep a record. We still have the sheet of paper with the results from 6:19 to 11:35. It was shortly before midnight when the heavy-duty pain meds were administered and Nicole took a well deserved break and a short nap.

Nicole had packed as much as possible in advance so I used the list from prenatal class to get my things together and we set off for the labour and delivery rooms at Loma Linda University Medical Center where we had been pre-registered. As soon as we arrived at the hospital things started to become a lot more difficult than we had imagined.

The first big challenge was actually being admitted to the hospital. I had been to hospitals in Canada before but the first major difference between the two opposing health care systems (US vs Canada) literally hit us in the face immediately. A very large VISA sign was pasted right onto the door. You do not get in unless you actually hand over your credit card. The fact that we had been pre-registered and had documented pre-authorized medical coverage was irrelevant.

We eventually got the admission all sorted and were escorted into the labour and delivery area where we were met by what can only be described as a slightly deranged nurse in charge of the labour rooms that night. When we described our situation with the high risk pregnancy due to the fetal diagnosis, her rather off-hand comment was, "Oh yeah, we get that here all the time, it usually turns out to be nothing." According to her the referring doctors got it wrong more often than not. We told her that we certainly would not have come all the way from northern Canada if we had not been at least reasonably certain of the diagnosis but she was having none of it. The only bit of good news that she did give us was that the high risk obstetrician who had been following the pregnancy for the last few weeks when Nicole had moved to California was on call that night and would be sleeping in the hospital.

We expected that perhaps the high-priced help might be stopping by to check on us but we did not see him until several hours after the actual delivery (many hours later) when he popped his head into Nicole's room to say hello. Instead we got a very, very tired looking resident who would not actually say when it was he had last slept – I think he had lost track and could not remember ever having slept. He was quite a nice young man and seemed to know what he was doing. He soon established that the baby's heart rate would drop every time Nicole had a contraction. We suggested that perhaps we should consult the obstetrician who apparently was in house and he agreed. He called and got the advice that Nicole should wear an oxygen mask. This seemed to alleviate the heart rate problem but caused a different dilemma. Now Nicole was attached to monitors and an oxygen source and the nurse insisted she be confined to her bed, unable to move around. I have never had contractions but I have been told by those who have that one of the worst positions to be in during this situation is flat on your back in bed. It is sort of like having a really, really bad Charley horse in your calf muscle when you are pinned down and can not move your leg to relieve the pain – only orders of magnitude worse and it goes on for hours on end. At one point things got so tense that Nicole insisted that she was leaving. It was all I could do to keep her from running out screaming – not that I wasn't considering it myself, but we were trapped.

Late in the evening we finally managed to convince the nurse that it was time for some serious pain medication and the anaesthetist came by and read Nicole her rights. She signed the consent form and he administered an epidural. To this day Nicole refers to him as her hero. She was able to take a break and managed to sleep for an hour or two during which time there was a shift change. It was like night and day. From then on we began to witness why Loma Linda hospital is considered to have a first-class neonatal program, second to none.

It was mid-morning the next day when we finally moved to the delivery room and two young female obstetricians took charge. They were fabulous and it was during one of the last big contractions that one of them reached over and pressed a red button on the side of the delivery table. Almost instantly six figures all dressed in grey surgical scrubs wearing matching masks which obscured their faces, each carrying a specific tool or instrument rushed in and stood in an orderly line at the foot of the delivery table.

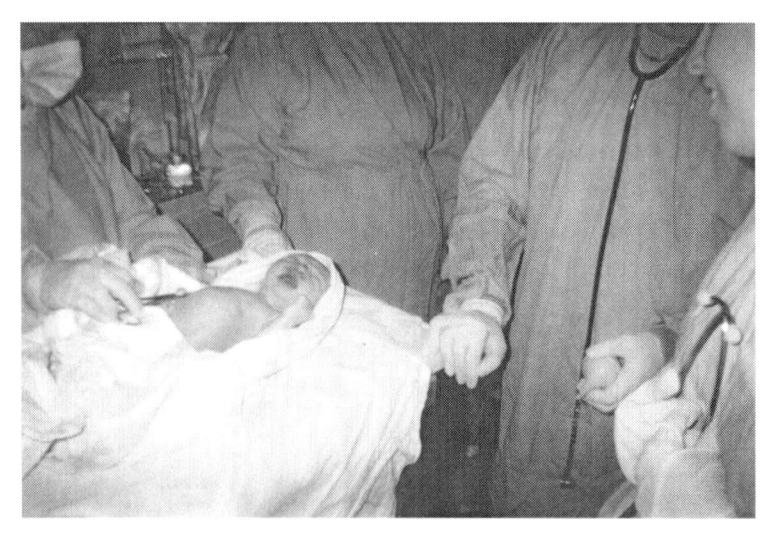

Mark – minutes after he was born – surrounded by the neonatal team

Nicole had had her eyes closed for a few seconds and when she opened them she looked over at me in shock and asked; "Who are they?" "I think they have come for the kid," I replied. With amazing proficiency the team went to work and within minutes they had the baby assessed and wrapped in a nice flannel blanket. Nicole insisted on holding him but they refused. They reluctantly handed him to me very briefly and I held him at her side for a few seconds. He opened his large eyes and stared up at us, his face filled with intensity and determination. From that brief look I got a huge boost of encouragement. It had been and would continue to be a long and arduous journey but I got the first inkling that maybe – just maybe - this decision to come to California was not all folly. For Nicole it was a major disappointment not to have been able to at least give him a hug. "What if he had actually died?" she would later say. That would have been tragic but fortunately he lives and we try to make up for that lack of an immediate mother's touch all the time.

Chapter 2
The binding of Isaac

"Take now thy son, thine only son Isaac, whom thou lovest, and get thee into the land of Moriah; and offer him there for a burnt offering upon one of the mountains which I will tell thee of."

God, *Genesis 22:2*

Once upon a time, according to a very old legend, a man called Abraham left the land of his father and mother and set off into the wilderness to find his fortune. He took with him a whole entourage including his wife Sarah, a woman of great beauty, his nephew Lot, as well as servants and herds and flocks for he did not intend to return. In fact he had been directed by divine insight that he would not only find a new home but that his descendants would establish a great nation. He encountered numerous difficulties on his search, in part because he had no fixed plan and no definite destination. He wandered around in the desert for longer than most of us have been alive.

His domestic situation was not very happy in part due to the fact that his wife's beauty was legendary. This was not an asset to him, but rather often a great detriment. At least once in his travels he lied about his relationship, pretending she was his sister, for fear her envious admirers would kill him. Their marriage was problematic for other reasons, as she also bore him no children. As they grew older she gave up on having any children and convinced him to take her female servant as a mate in order to produce descendants for the new homeland. As might be expected this plan did not go well and the world is still trying to sort out the consequences.

According to the legend Sarah was well past menopause when one evening Abraham suggested, guided once again by divine inspiration, that they "lie together" in the hopes that she might bear him a son who would establish the great nation of his dreams. One can only imagine her response, but this encounter did in fact result in a child – a son called Isaac. Finally everything seemed to be coming together for Abraham. He had found the homeland he was searching for and he had a son through whom he might father a great nation. However, it was just then that God directed him to sacrifice Isaac on a mountain in that land known as Moriah.

It was to this mountain that Abraham travelled with Isaac when he was still a boy and they built an altar. Abraham then took his son whom he loved dearly, his heir – the future father of the descendants he was convinced he would have - and laid him on the altar and was about to stab him to death as a human sacrifice. Fortunately for everyone involved, there was a direct divine intervention at this point and an animal was provided and sacrificed in Isaac's stead.

Throughout history, this act, referred to as 'the binding of Isaac,' has fascinated everyone who would ponder its meaning. The great thinkers of the ages have tried to make some sense of this story. Painters, sculptors, poets, musicians, playwrights, philosophers, and theologians have struggled to understand the binding of Isaac. The earliest recorded artistic work depicting this story is a mosaic of floor panels crafted in the 6th century in a synagogue in Beit Alpha. The work is attributed to an artisan, Marianos, and his son Hanina. In recent times Leonard Cohen's Story of Isaac, Soren Kierkegaard's *Fear and Trembling*, and Chagall's Sacrifice of Isaac are some of my personal favourite studies of the subject. For me, each work always raises more questions than it answers.

The binding of Isaac was in fact Abraham's defining act. He had done a lot of crazy things in his life but it was because of Mount Moriah more than anything else that he became the father of three of the world's great religions. Many of us have left our homes in search of our fortune; many of us have borne the consequences of choosing a spouse of great beauty; too many of us have agonized over childless partnerships; but who among us would even contemplate taking one of our children whom we dearly love, binding them and attempting to drive a knife through their heart as an act of human sacrifice? Such an act is so horrible that we cannot even imagine it occurring in our real day-to-day lives, much less doing it ourselves. In fact it is so incredible that most of us prefer not to think about it, dismissing it as a crazy notion not worth contemplating or desperately trying to escape having to ponder too long such a thought.

There are in fact many ways to lose a child. Some are an indirect or even a direct result of what we have done or left undone. But these are not quite the same as taking it upon ourselves to end our child's life by our own hand. On rare occasions parents must, however, make life or death decisions for their children and this was how my own journey to Mount Moriah started.

Chapter 3
Anfechtung

"Therefore if Abraham would express himself in terms of the universal, he must say that his situation is a temptation (Anfechtung), for he has no higher expression for that universal which stands above the universal which he transgresses."

Kierkegaard, *Fear and Trembling*

My first exposure to Abraham's story was as a young boy in Sunday school. There was a long row of reprints of classical paintings depicting Biblical themes all along the top of one wall. If you have ever been to Sunday school you know the sort of stuff: the last supper, the crucifixion, Moses parting the Red Sea, and so on. At the end of the row was the binding of Isaac by one of the early classical painters and as is often characteristic of their work, the use of light draws one to the focal point of the picture: in this case, Abraham's face. His face was at once beautiful and horrible - if that is possible - and that look has stayed with me all these years.

As a student in philosophy class, I had read *Fear and Trembling* in which the author, Kierkegaard analyzes the binding of Isaac in great depth. Later in life I re-read the book several times until I thought that I understood it at least on an academic level. I listened to Dylan's *Highway 61 Revisited* and Leonard Cohen's *Story of Isaac*, and I had had long and heated discussions about the binding of Isaac with other young students and professors at university. In spite of all this I was still, like so many others, avoiding the real and difficult questions raised by the legend, usually dismissing the whole myth as too bizarre and gruesome to take too seriously, preferring rather to look at it from the armchair of philosophy. That is until one day I was confronted with a situation from which it was impossible to run – even the most sophisticated avoidance tactics were not going to work. I experienced *anfechtung* for myself.

It all started following a visit to our family medical clinic in Saskatchewan. Nicole and I had recently finished our studies at Queen's University in Ontario and had moved halfway across the country to Saskatoon. She was about six months pregnant when we moved and had been getting early prenatal care at the student medical clinic on campus. Our doctor had been very pleased to be working with us because she didn't get many young women at the University clinic who were pregnant and actually did not want to terminate the pregnancy – in fact we were her first prenatal case. We had been doing everything right. We had gone for regular visits and had had an ultrasound done at eleven weeks. Like many first-time parents, we treasured the grainy photos we were given of our child. We put them up on the refrigerator; Nicole painted several artistic impressions of them which we proudly displayed in our apartment. We were convinced that the child was a girl and we gave her a name: Meg.

When we got to Saskatoon we had been referred to a new physician, an acquaintance of our doctor in Ontario and armed with the appropriate files we went for our first visit as soon as we had settled in. Everything seemed to be fine with one minor exception – in the file the doctor in Ontario had actually calculated two different due dates two weeks apart and it was unclear which one was correct. We didn't think this was a problem but our new doctor insisted that because this was our first child she would like to have a definite idea as to the correct date so she ordered another ultrasound.

I was not able to accompany Nicole to this second ultrasound but I stopped by to pick her up. As soon as I saw her coming out of the building I knew there was a problem. We had expected some new photos for the gallery but the technician had been very abrupt, even unfriendly. Each time Nicole had asked to see the images on the monitor she was told it was not convenient to let her do so. She was worried – something was wrong. I tried to stay calm and suggested that perhaps the technician was just having a bad day.

★★★

One day later our doctor called us and asked us to come in to discuss the ultrasound report. Nicole had been right, there was definitely something very wrong. They had observed a large mass associated with the child's heart and although the physician writing the report suggested an evaluation be done postpartum our doctor was having none of it. We needed to check the problem out right away. She had made an appointment with the paediatric cardiologist at the University hospital for the next day. Although I remained hopeful that there was no need for grave concern, Nicole was not convinced. "These specialists are busy people," she said, "one can wait months to see them. You don't just get an appointment the next day unless something is seriously wrong."

When we got to the hospital for our appointment the next day we were immediately ushered into an ultrasound room. Soon after starting the scan, the technician called in an elderly man who introduced himself as a cardiac surgeon. He studied the monitor intently and very quickly called one of his colleagues who came in with several of his assistants. Introductions and handshakes were not happening at this point. It didn't take long before there were approximately ten people all huddled around the monitor, staring at it, at times muttering to each other and nodding.

It was surreal for us because Nicole was lying on the examination table and I was sitting on her left side at the front of the room. The monitor was on the right hand side at the bottom of the room. Our only connection to the group was via a cord that connected the probe on Nicole's abdomen to the machine in the corner. Everyone's attention was focused on the monitor on the other side of the room, which we could not see - we could only see the backs of the people in the huddle. It was as if the group didn't realize we were actually in room. We could not really make out what they were saying all the time but at one point we did clearly hear someone say that they did not see a left ventricle and several others agreed.

This went on for what seemed like an eternity until the elderly man who had come in first, who seemed to be the leader, spoke to the group and said, "So we are all in agreement then?" to which everyone nodded and started to disperse as rapidly as they had appeared. The leader then turned to us and said, "Well I guess that is all. We will contact your family doctor and she will explain everything to you."

Both Nicole and I were already somewhat shell-shocked by the whole scene involving the huddle around the monitor but we were absolutely stunned by this comment. We both had taken enough biology in university to know that a left ventricle was rather essential to the human circulatory system. Did they think we had not heard them? Did they think we did not understand the severity of this diagnosis? I immediately confronted the surgeon and told him that his suggestion regarding waiting to see the family doctor was highly inappropriate (though I can assure you I did not phrase it quite that diplomatically). He glanced at his colleague who was one of the few people still in the room and then suggested that perhaps we should all go to his office.

When we got to the office the two senior cardiologists informed us that our child had what is known as hypoplastic left heart syndrome. With the aid of illustrations and models they explained to us that in this situation the left ventricle does not develop – this was in fact the mass of tissue attached to the heart referred to in the ultrasound report. They went on to explain that as long as the child stays in the uterus there is no problem. The left ventricle normally pumps blood from the lungs and then through the aorta to the entire body, providing a supply of oxygen to the tissues and maintaining blood pressure.

However, in utero the lungs are not used. Oxygen is supplied by the mother's circulation via the umbilical cord. The blood does not actually go to the lungs of the foetus to pick up oxygen but rather the pulmonary arteries are connected to the pulmonary veins in the foetal circulatory system.

Most of the blood detours past the lungs from the right ventricle through the ductus arteriosis, a foetal arch, and back to the left ventricle and then the aorta. If the left ventricle is missing you have a three-chambered heart and *in utero* the right ventricle maintains the blood pressure and pumps the foetal blood throughout the body of the foetus. With hypoplastic left heart syndrome the problem only becomes apparent and critical at birth, when the ductus arteriosis is re-absorbed and the circulation to the lungs is necessary to sustain a supply of oxygen to the body. Without the foetal arch and a left ventricle, blood pressure in the body cannot be maintained and blood begins to accumulate in the lungs because the right ventricle is pumping blood in but there is no way to move the blood out.

After a very long and relatively calm discussion, Nicole asked the obvious question, front and centre in both our minds, "What do we need to do to deal with this problem?" Both of us expected that there would be an explanation of some surgery or treatment forthcoming at this point. The answer was however one of the strangest bits of medical-speak I think I have ever heard: *This condition is not compatible with life.*

The time it takes for the foetal arch to degenerate is quite variable but once it does the newborn will soon suffocate and die. This was the surgeon's original guarded response to the question, but neither Nicole nor I were happy with this answer and when we pressed the surgeons for more information they did tell us about two alternatives. Both alternatives were at that time highly experimental. One was a cardiac transplant at or shortly after birth, and the other was reconstructive surgery known as the Norwood procedure.

The Norwood procedure was being used in the central and eastern USA to treat hypoplastic left heart and required several open heart surgeries within the first two years of the child's life. At the time the success rate was poor. The child would be left with a relatively inefficient three-chambered heart with the right ventricle serving as the only pump while blood carrying oxygen from the lungs would constantly mix with blood low in oxygen coming from the body.

Infant heart transplants, our second option, were being pioneered by Dr. Lenard Bailey at Loma Linda Medical Center in California. The biggest problem with this option was that often a donor was not found in time to perform the transplant. Even if it was - and if the transplant was then successful - the child would have to live with foreign tissue, making the use of anti-rejection drugs mandatory. Not only would there always be a threat of rejection, but these drugs suppress the immune system which could result in many other complications like increased risk of infections and cancer.

★★★

It was late in the evening when we finally left the hospital. The surgeons had photocopied a lot of information regarding both the Norwood and transplant procedures for us to look over at home. They told us we were actually very lucky because this condition was usually only diagnosed at birth when the parents had very little time to think about any treatment options. At least we had time, they said, but that did little to relieve the agony of making the decision. In hindsight they were definitely right, time *was* a valuable commodity.

The next day our family doctor called us and we went in to see her. She gave us a lot more information and suggested we have a whole set of tests done to ensure that our child was actually a candidate for treatment. If there were any other health-related issues they might preclude any treatment at all and in that case we could spare ourselves the stress of trying to decide what to do. So it was off to the hospital almost every day for the next week for the first of what would be several amniocenteses and many other scans and tests. We were also given a list of contacts in the eastern USA and California, hospital personnel who could give us advice as well as some parents whose children had be treated for hypoplastic left heart.

The stress level was almost unbearable; coming and going to hospital, calling complete strangers to talk about very personal issues and the whole time trying to decide what was the right thing to do. One afternoon we had some free time so we went out for a late lunch. Some of my new colleagues at work whom I was meeting for the first time were going to join us. We thought it would be a good idea to discuss something other than the problem at hand. Nicole and I had arrived early and were standing in the parking lot outside the restaurant. We kept going over our problem asking the same questions over and over – why was this happening to us? What had we done to deserve this? Why couldn't anyone seem to help us? At one point Nicole suggested an answer to our questions; "Maybe this is some sort of a test to see how much we really love this child?" At that moment I finally understood – this was *anfechtung*.

I had read several different translations of Kierkegaard's Fear and Trembling and in each translation *anfechtung* had a slightly different meaning: a test, a challenge, a temptation, a struggle. None of the translators seemed to be comfortable with one single English word, in fact one of the best translations had simply declared the word untranslatable and had just used the German.

I had become functionally literate in German while studying in Gottingen and I thought I understood the word. *Fechten* means to duel with swords - *anfechtung* then would mean to challenge someone to a duel. Considering that I have absolutely no swashbuckling experience whatsoever being challenged to a duel would certainly be a life-threatening experience, but even that idea did not quite compete with real *anfechtung* when I encountered it. *Anfechtung* is in fact the mother of all personal challenges or struggles - a test which rocks you to the very core of your being. It is both life-altering and life-affirming.

Chapter 4
Infinite resignation
– the last stage prior to faith

"In the infinite resignation there is peace and rest."
"The infinite resignation is the last stage prior to faith, so that one who has not made this movement has not faith; for only in the infinite resignation do I become clear to myself with respect to my eternal validity, and only then can there be any question of grasping existence by virtue of faith."
"Faith therefore is not an aesthetic emotion but something far higher, precisely because it has resignation as its presupposition; it is not an immediate instinct of the heart, but is the paradox of life and existence."

Kierkegaard, *Fear and Trembling*

So you have just been challenged to the very core of your being and the first movement you must make is resignation. For a long time I did not understand this response to *anfechtung*. It seemed to me that any human being worth his salt should stand up and fight after experiencing *anfechtung*. I could not make the distinction between resignation and giving up. I had seen lots of people who had given up: on themselves, on society, on life. One only needs to walk the streets of any major city and really look into the faces of people passing by to see examples of what happens when someone gives up. The same people walk by each other at the same place every day but do not seem to notice their surroundings. It is as if they are on treadmills, going through the motions of their days automatically. They do not appear to be in distress and there is no sense of desperation about them, but their faces are empty and expressionless. There is no spring in their step and there is no joy in their demeanour. They are living unhappy lives with no meaning, following routines without fulfilment. How could this possibly be an appropriate response to *anfechtung*?

The night I began to understand the difference between giving up and resignation I was sitting in a small room in Loma Linda University Medical Centre. The room was a lounge outside the infant intensive care unit where Mark, our seven-day-old son, lay dying with a malfunctioning heart. It was late in the evening and the team of cardiac surgeons had called Nicole and me in for a meeting. They were looking noticeably tired as they had just returned from a hospital where a sixteen-month-old girl had died; they had been given permission to harvest her heart. They had transported it in a cooler back to Loma Linda and were preparing to transplant this heart into Mark's chest.

It had been a day of intense emotion and drama. In the morning we had been to visit Mark in the intensive care unit. He seemed to be getting weaker and we noticed that the colour in his face was draining away more every day. After a relatively short visit we left and had spent most of the day with another couple from Canada. We had originally met them only several days earlier at the hospital the night their daughter received her heart transplant to treat the same condition Mark had. Tragically, the transplant had not worked in their case. Their daughter died about a week after her surgery. She never left the intensive care unit of the hospital.

We helped this couple pack up their belongings in the small apartment they had rented across the street from the hospital. Most of their things consisted of the equipment and clothing needed to care for a newborn infant – painful reminders to us all. We cried a lot. When we finished packing all their things into our car, we went out for lunch and then we drove them to a funeral home out in the desert near Loma Linda to collect one last item - a small urn containing the ashes of their baby girl. We cried a lot more as we drove them to the airport to fly home.

It was late afternoon when Nicole and I returned to our apartment from the airport and although we did not speak about it, I knew both of us were thinking that we might have made a grave error coming to Loma Linda in search of a miracle. I don't think I have ever been more despondent and I was certainly was very close to giving up. We knew we should be getting ready to go in for our evening visit to see Mark but neither of us had the energy to make that happen and we were both dreading having to go back to the intensive care unit. Then, at the very darkest moment of our struggle, the phone rang. Nicole answered it. At first the conversation sounded like idle chatter but then suddenly there was an edgy excitement in Nicole's voice. She hung up the phone and breathlessly informed me that they had a donor for Mark and that if we wanted to see him before he went into surgery we would need to hurry.

We rushed into the hospital's paediatric intensive care unit and found that Mark had been moved to a special area for preparation. From a distance it appeared that there was a flurry of activity around him but when we were allowed into the area we saw that the lights had been dimmed and all the individuals working on him seemed relaxed and calm. They had started to chill his body and he was wearing a little blue and white striped toque – fitting attire given his Canadian roots. We were not able to pick him up and hold him but I squeezed his little fingers hard before we had to go.

We waited anxiously for several hours to meet with the surgeons before they started the operation and it was late in the evening when we finally were asked to come to the small lounge outside the intensive care unit. The meeting actually went on for quite some time because we were required to carefully read several documents outlining the risks involved with the surgery as well as many other legal forms. It was the kind of stuff you often don't read before clicking the "I accept" tab on your computer. At one point while we were speaking with the surgeons, I found myself thinking, "This is crazy, there are so many ways this can go wrong, how could we possibly imagine that this is a good idea?"

Eventually, we were asked to sign and initial the relevant forms giving our permission for the team to remove our son's heart and replace it with the donor's.

As we were signing the forms I experienced a feeling I had never felt before, and I was euphoric. It was not desperation and it was certainly not giving up, even though I felt like I was giving *everything* up. It was resignation. We had finalized the decision and there was no turning back. We would need to repeat this moment of resignation over and over again during Mark's life. Although my hand faltered as I signed my name, it felt as if a huge weight was being lifted from my shoulders: at last, peace and rest.

Chapter 5
An Un-ethical Decision

If the end brings me out all right, what is said against me won't amount to anything. If the end brings me out wrong, ten angels swearing I was right would make no difference.

Abraham Lincoln

Some decisions we must make are difficult because there seems to be an infinite number of possibilities, while others are difficult because there is no course of action which is obviously right. When we were struggling with our decision in Saskatoon following our son's diagnosis, there were really only two choices, but this did not make our decision any easier. Either we would decide to seek medical intervention to correct Mark's hypoplastic left heart, or we would let our child die shortly after his birth. If we chose medical intervention, then we'd have to choose what kind. There were only two medical centers in the world offering procedures to correct the condition – one on the eastern sea-board of the USA where Dr. Norwood had pioneered the procedure bearing his name, and the other was a transplant shortly after birth at Loma Linda Medical Center in California.

At the outset I was sure that given enough information I would come to the right decision. I would rely on my scientific training – I did after all have a Ph.D. in science. Nicole and I went to the library and read everything we could find on the Norwood procedure and infant heart transplants. As both procedures were basically in the experimental stages, there was not that much information regarding the long-term outcome of either.

The Norwood procedure would require three open heart surgeries within the first five years of the child's life. Essentially, a three-chambered heart was constructed using the right ventricle and right and left atria, thereby restoring heart function in spite of the fact that the left ventricle was missing. Each of the surgeries had a published survival rate which was somewhere near the 80% range at that time. If one were to take a rigorous statistical approach, he could conclude that the child has approximately a 50% chance of survival. (Using the Product Rule in statistics, .8 cubed is 51%). However, we also needed to take quality of life into consideration. Not only would we subject our child to three rather serious surgical interventions but in the end he would have a three-chambered heart which works perfectly well in a frog or other amphibian (which needs to be able to breathe under water as well as on dry land) but in a human being not so much. Oxygen-rich blood coming from the lungs would constantly mix with blood with low oxygen levels in the single ventricle making the supply of oxygen to the body very inefficient. The end effect on the quality of life for the child was not yet well documented.

An infant transplant would involve only one dramatic surgical procedure (although there are patients who required and survived several transplants). The survival rate was estimated at approximately 80% at that time, but one also had to take into consideration that in only approximately 65% of the cases was a donor organ found in time. Once again from a purely statistical standpoint, the chances of success were about 50% (.8 times .65 equals 52%). Quality of life post-transplant was highly variable, with some children doing very well and others struggling with a range of chronic medical issues. The life expectancy of a person post-transplant was estimated at 12 years, but we were assured that with the infant transplants the estimate might be slightly more optimistic. It was thought that if the foreign organ was placed in the recipient early enough in life the chance of rejection by the host immune system would be a lot lower. Rejection of the heart was in fact the single most important factor that would determine the quality of our child's life. Transplant patients need to take medications to suppress their immune system so they do not reject the transplanted organ which is foreign to them. These medications increase their risk of developing cancer, as another function of the immune system is to seek and destroy pre-cancerous cells in the body. The drugs also have various other undesirable side effects such as kidney damage and increased susceptibility to microbial infections, among other things. The severity of the side effects would really depend on the level of medication required to suppress rejection. If one was fortunate and the donor organ was a good match - thereby lowering the risk of rejection - the level of medication required could be kept relatively low and the side effects would be minimal.

I very quickly came to the conclusion that there was no preferred course of action based on the scientific evidence available at the time, and the ethical issues related to our decision began to become rather important. By deciding against medical intervention we were sentencing our child to certain death very shortly after he was born. Deciding in favour of medical intervention might be sentencing him to a very unhappy existence, in which he would be a sickly individual seriously handicapped in terms of living a meaningful life and constantly struggling with health issues. So although the alternatives were limited the outcomes, at least in the case of intervention, were ambiguous. For a week I was almost constantly troubled by two different nightmares. In one dream I had decided against intervention and some years later I was walking through a playground. A group of young children were playing and someone pointed out that one of them had been born with hypoplastic left heart and had undergone surgery. She was now happily getting on with life. Wouldn't that be wonderful?

In the second dream I kept envisioning our child lying in a hospital bed kept alive with the aid of advanced medical technology. He was unable to go outside to join the other children in the playground. He had been sentenced to an unhappy existence in hospital, constantly struggling for survival and perhaps then dying before getting the chance to really enjoy life.

Another ethical consideration which also concerned me was the cost of intervention. Was it really fair that we could spend hundreds of thousands of dollars to keep our child alive when around the world other children were dying because they did not have access to clean water and medications and vaccines which would cost only a few dollars to supply? Most of us try our best to do the right thing especially when it concerns the welfare of our own children. But I feel it is also important that we do the right thing for the right reasons. Sometimes we do the right thing for the wrong reasons and at times we might even be obliged to do the wrong thing for the right reasons. Careful consideration of all the ethical issues involved also led me no closer to deciding the right course of action. The nightmares haunted me. In the end Nicole and I came to the decision to proceed with the transplant. This decision was based more on intuition than anything else. Fortunately, we both came to the same decision.

It was some time later that I came to the realization that neither science nor ethics could bring us to a decision in this particular case. While we were living near the hospital I was able to work in a research lab on campus at Loma Linda. When parents of children with hypoplastic left heart were visiting the Center trying to make a decision either for or against a transplant, they would often call me to discuss their decision. I have to say that I was somewhat biased in favour of transplant after Mark's brilliant recovery and progress. In one particular case I met with a young couple and spoke to them for a long time about our experience and the complexity of arriving at a decision. Several days later I was speaking to one of the transplant coordinators and she told me that the couple had decided against intervention. I must have been visibly upset because I thought they would have been excellent candidates for the transplant program. Noticing that I was upset, the nurse told me that many parents decided against a transplant for a variety of reasons, all of which were valid for them. Some already had a family and moving to California would involve a major cost as well as being a major upheaval for the family. Some just didn't believe that it is the best course of action. I came to understand that in fact there was no right or wrong decision in this case, and therefore it becomes a decision which is outside the realm of ethics. There is no way to make a rational decision based on scientific evidence either; the decision would have to be made on faith alone.

Chapter 6

Let Nature take its course

When it all comes down to dust
I will kill you if I must
I will help you if I can
When it all comes down to dust
I will help you if I must
I will kill you if I can

Leonard Cohen, *Story of Isaac*

Traditionally childbirth and neonatal care has been women's work. Young mothers, assisted by their grandmothers, mothers, and aunties, would use their collective knowledge and instincts to bring new life into the world and then to nurture that little bundle of joy. This type of maternal joint venture is something we share with many of the large mammals. I am going to go out on a somewhat precarious limb for someone of my gender and say that this is probably the way it should be.

The male of the species lacks some of the essential equipment required for the process. Oh, we can perform several of the simpler tasks of neonatal care. I thoroughly enjoyed holding my babies for hours, rocking them gently while softly singing to them the traditional hymns, lullabies, and always including at least several Dylan tunes for their edification. I also really enjoyed giving them their baths, one of my favourite tasks of all time. I even found that changing their diapers was quite rewarding. It was a little gross while I was doing it but I felt all clean and wholesome when I had finished.

For the big stuff though, they needed their Mom. I was constantly reminded of this whenever I found myself frantically dashing around the kitchen with a frozen baggie of milk or formula stuffed into my armpit, desperately wishing the water would boil, or fiddling with a can opener and baby bottles, the whole time accompanied by the baby shrieking blue murder to my own expletive lyrics. I must say that I am envious that their mother could come along and quietly and instantaneously deal with the issue. I am, however, not envious of some of the other required equipment. At least once a month I say a little prayer of thanks that I do not possess an organ in my abdomen which sloughs off its internal membrane, the messy business known in the vernacular as "getting my period." The same holds true for having that same organ which violently and uncontrollably contracts during delivery – NO, NO, NO, thank you very much. My own small part in the reproductive process was so much more fun, especially getting to practice.

Over the course of the last century the role of mothers and grandmothers in childbirth and child care began to diminish. Various members of the medical community started to get very involved in childbirth and neonatal care. At first this would be the family doctor, but later two major branches of medicine - obstetrics and paediatrics - evolved. Pregnancy and childbirth came to be viewed as a medical condition or intervention rather than something which occurred naturally. It was in the 1960s and 70s that some women started to rebel. They realized that they had given up a great deal of control and power in a significant portion of motherhood. Together with some of the grandmothers and aunties they started to demand it back.

At about the same time medical technology was advancing at an unprecedented rate. Treatment for premature birth and many developmental defects became not only feasible but normalized; in many cases parents began to expect and even demand miracles. A variety of issues all came to a head at the same time in what could be considered a perfect storm with some colossal ethical, moral, and legal clashes in the 1980s and '90s. Minor skirmishes quickly escalated into major battles involving questions pertaining to life and death issues like when to offer or withhold treatment or when to discontinue treatment in cases where the outcomes where highly uncertain. In many situations it was impossible to predict the likelihood of a disaster or a miracle. These battles occurred between doctors and mothers, doctors and fathers, mothers and fathers, doctors and doctors. The politicians, lawyers, and ultimately the accountants got involved because we, collectively, quickly found that medical intervention was a very costly undertaking. What had traditionally been the domain of the mothers in our society had become a very complex business indeed.

It was within this storm of controversy that Nicole and I had to make our decision as to whether or not to seek medical intervention to save the life of our unborn child. Although we got excellent medical advice regarding possible interventions, we were constantly amazed that there appeared to be little advice on the moral and ethical implications of making a decision not to intervene. Actually it was absolutely shocking how the decision *not* to intervene in hypoplastic left heart syndrome was being handled. On several occasions we were told that we could just take our baby home and let nature take its course – and that was it.

On the surface it sounded like the natural and beautiful thing to do, a kinder and gentler approach. Luckily we spoke with families who had at least initially decided in favour of this option. Can you imagine what that must have been like, especially for a first-time mother? Each time she would put her infant down for a nap she would agonize over the fact that he would likely not wake up. She would watch in absolute dread as her baby very slowly and painfully suffocated to death. In some cases the families who chose this option were absolutely devastated within hours of arriving at home and desperately tried to reverse their decision. I was horrified by the thought that we might take our baby home and watch it die. It was when Nicole and I had spoken to the mothers who had done this that it became very clear to both of us that letting nature take its course in our home was not an option. In the "good old days" when the grandmothers and aunties were in charge there was no other option, but there was also no prior knowledge of certain death. In some ways things were much simpler then but in many ways they were also much, much more difficult. Sometimes babies died shortly after birth.

From my experiences growing up on a farm with animals that were both companions and a source of income, I was no stranger to death and suffering. To watch an animal that we valued or even loved, which was facing certain death, linger on and suffer was definitely not tolerated. We made every effort to end life as humanely and quickly as possible in situations where death was inevitable. For me the suggestion that we would sit at home watching and waiting without any mention of palliative care for the infant and no support for the parents seemed incredibly callous – absolutely philistine.

Now, over a decade into the new millennium, the dust has started to settle on many of the battles involving birth, as well as neonatal and palliative care. Hopefully we will find a balance which will allow mothers as well as elders to reclaim control over their traditional rights and still maintain state-of-the-art medical treatment. However we must abandon euphemistic terminology and the notion that Mother Nature is always kind and gentle – only giving us life. She is also intimately involved with death, which is often violent, premature and unfair. We must remember that science and technology can enhance the quality and sustainability of life but they do not trump our basic instincts and intuitive wisdom.

Chapter 7
Just a little too BIG

"It's just a little too big but don't worry, he'll grow into it."

Dr. S. Gundry, paediatric cardiac surgeon, Loma Linda University Medical Center, about Mark's new heart.

The neonatal intensive care unit at Loma Linda University Medical Center is a large rectangular room which can accommodate approximately 60 infants. It is an open space with individual stations arranged in neat rows across the width of the room. If one looks out over the unit during the day he would see several teams of medical specialists including physicians, fellows, interns, and medical students checking on babies with a wide variety of medical disorders. One will also see many parents with their babies because they were encouraged to spend as much time with their newborns as possible.

This is where we waited for a donor organ to come available. In fact all the babies waiting for a heart transplant were in this room, not grouped together but scattered about throughout the unit. In spite of that we very quickly got to know the other parents of the babies waiting. News of an additional baby arriving at Loma Linda awaiting a heart transplant spread quickly through the group of parents and the new parents were immediately accepted into the very close-knit group. We were all going through a very dramatic shared experience which brought us all together.

I was not entirely comfortable in this group. We were all waiting for exactly the same thing. Transplantation of organs in newborns did not require the complex process of tissue matching that is necessary for adults. The theory is that the human immune system does not begin to develop until after birth occurs. It is the immune system that recognizes cells which are foreign to the body and mounts an attack which causes the rejection of the donor organ. If the donor organ is introduced while the immune system is developing there is much less risk that it will be rejected because it will be recognized as self. This means that any newborn can use almost every organ which comes available.

There were approximately ten babies waiting for a heart in that room at Loma Linda. My concern was if a donor came available, which baby would get it? The answer was never made clear to us. Was it the baby who had been waiting the longest? Some babies tolerated waiting with a hypoplastic left heart better than others. There was a rumour that if a particular baby needed a transplant more urgently than others who had been waiting longer, the more urgent case would go ahead. But every case was urgent. Every day the babies were waiting their immune systems were developing. At what time point did tissue matching start to become necessary? There was no clear answer to this question but it had been suggested that the optimal window for transplantation was within approximately two weeks after birth. There were babies who waited for more than two months for a donor. Did this mean that they would not do as well later on?

The ticking immune systems' clocks were not the only cause for concern. With each passing day the babies with defective hearts were becoming more and more listless. Because they were functioning with a three-chambered heart their blood pressure was declining. Their skin colour was becoming paler and more sallow looking. In fact there were a number of reasons why all the parents waiting for a donor for their babies wanted to get one as soon as possible. Perhaps the most important issue was that we were all very aware of the fact that at the time only approximately sixty percent of those waiting would actually get a donor heart. It was for this reason more than any other that I felt particularly uneasy within the group of other parents with babies waiting. Who was going to decide which of these babies would live and which would die?

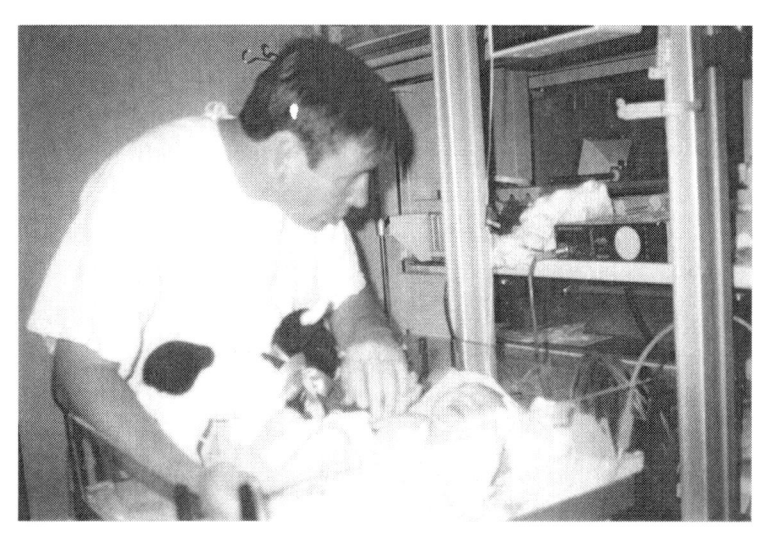

Mark in intensive care waiting for a donor heart. I became obsessed with monitoring his blood oxygen levels.

Exactly one week after Mark was born a young girl with type A blood died, and her heart was healthy and available for donation. Although a tissue match was not relevant with the babies, blood type was important. All the other waiting babies were blood type O – Mark was the only baby with blood type A waiting. The other babies could only use a heart which came from an individual with O blood type. And so, quite miraculously, Mark had a new heart only one week after he was born.

We were allowed to see Mark the morning after his transplant. He was in a small room at one end of the neonatal intensive care unit – a kind of very intensive care unit. When we went in there were three nurses surrounding his small bed and the number of cables attached to Mark's little body had increased 10-fold after his operation. We had been told that he would look much better after his operation because his colour would improve. His skin did have a healthy rosy colour but his head seemed to be swollen and he had two tubes coming out of his chest draining blood. One of the nurses was constantly banging on these tubes with a piece of wood to dislodge the clots. She suggested we could help her. I declined. Another nurse was continually monitoring Mark's vital signs: heart rate, blood pressure, blood oxygen levels, breathing rate, etc. It was very intense but we spent at least 18 hours a day with Mark for the first few days and we quickly started to notice changes. Because he had been on a heart bypass machine his kidneys had stopped working. Apparently one of the first positive signs that everything is progressing as it should is that the patient starts to pass urine after being on the machine. Within 12 hours of his operation Mark started to pee and then there was no end to wet diapers. The whole hospital seemed to have been informed of this event. I would be in the cafeteria and complete strangers would approach me and tell me how great it was that Mark had peed. The demeanour of the teams of specialists rounding on Mark grew less guarded and more relaxed, first by the hour and then by the day. The baby who was in the post-op room with him had a few complications which took longer to sort out so the change for us was quite obvious. The physicians, interns, and students would be laughing and joking about Mark's appearance but when they moved to the other side of the room they became more serious and the concern showed on their faces. The number of nurses for Mark quickly went from three to two, then down to one, who after the first two days just checked in from the larger room next door or as she was dealing with the other baby in the room.

It was when we first spoke with Dr. Gundry, the surgeon who had performed the operation, that we learned something about the donor we had not expected. Mark's donor was not an infant but rather a sixteen month old child. This meant that the heart he'd received was much bigger than an infant heart. At birth, the heart is approximately as big as a walnut but it grows quite quickly. In spite of the fact that Mark was a large baby the heart was actually much too big for his chest. To this day he holds some dubious world record for the ratio of size of donor to recipient in a heart transplant. The first thing the surgeon had said to us after the operation was, "It's just a little too big but don't worry, he'll grow into it." I immediately remembered growing up in a large family and getting hand-me-down clothes and boots from older siblings. That is exactly what my Mother had said to us when we complained about the fact that our "new" stuff didn't really fit. What kind of parents were we? We couldn't even get a heart that really fit him – his was much too big for his chest.

The fact that the heart was squished into the chest affected the way the heart beat and the age of the heart affected the rate. An older heart beats much more slowly. Right after birth the rate is really very rapid but as the heart increases in size, the rate at which it beats slows dramatically. This caused considerable problems for the teams of specialists. One team was the cardiologists who came around several times a day. They would listen to Mark's heart and check all the monitors. Their position regarding his heart rate was that the donor heart was very large so with each beat would pump more blood; therefore, the slow heart rate was ok. Next the team from general pediatrics would come around to check the monitors and listen to Mark's chest. They were concerned about the rate – yes the heart was bigger but the fact that it was squished inside the chest made it less efficient and therefore it still needed to beat faster. The groups rarely rounded at the same time so the problem persisted for several days until after the first week, a meeting of the entire group - 30 or so people - took place in the room with us present. The discussion about the heart rate was actually quite heated at times with the cardiologists insisting everything was ok and the pediatricians arguing that there was a problem. In the end they decided to attach yet another set of cables to Mark in order to control a pacemaker so they could regulate the heart rate artificially. It was a compromised solution and like so many compromises it didn't really work that well in real life. Now the team of cardiologists would arrive at Mark's bed and immediately fly into a panic - "Why is his heart beating so fast? Who turned up this pacemaker?" They would make the necessary adjustments and move on, Mark's heart beating a cool 85 beats per minute. Not long after the pediatricians would arrive and immediately turn up the pacemaker muttering abuse at the cardiologists under their breath. This pattern repeated itself for the rest of Mark's time in the hospital.

Another problem we had during the first week, post-op, had to do with feeding Mark. While the babies were waiting for donors, the staff encouraged the moms to feed them breast milk, though the weight and volume of everything going into and out of the babies had to be very closely monitored. Therefore the mothers needed to use a breast pump and store milk in labelled containers in a fridge in the intensive care unit so the nurses could access it at feeding time and feed only a very specific amount. At times the place seemed to be more of a milking parlour on a dairy farm than an intensive care facility. As parents we would get to bottle feed the infants ourselves if we were visiting at feeding time. We were very happy that several days after the operation one of the nurses suggested we discuss the possibility of breast feeding with the team. Once again there was a major disagreement within the larger group – some thought that it was too early not to be monitoring milk intake, others suggested that most babies who had become accustomed to bottle feeding would no longer accept the breast because they had to work harder at getting the milk out. We finally convinced everyone to let Nicole give it a try and if it really did not work out we would continue with the pumping and bottles. That afternoon the nurse noticed Nicole was getting ready to start breastfeeding and there was an immediate panic alert. Several more nurses came rushing in: "What was she thinking? You don't just suddenly start breastfeeding your baby." We were a little puzzled, thinking that maybe Mark had to be weighed before or after feeding. No, that was not the problem. Nicole had not actually watched the breastfeeding training video prior to proceeding. I made some derisory comment about us being mammals and would that not be an instinctive behaviour for human females? As my punishment for suggesting something so preposterous, I was forced to watch the video with her before she was allowed to start. After a few minutes and with a lot of coaching from a team of special nurses who had gathered for the event (none of whom had actually breast fed a baby themselves) Mark took to the breast and never looked back.

Exactly ten days after his operation it was suggested that we start to prepare to take Mark home. This was indeed good news not only because it meant that he was doing very well, but also because it allowed us to get out of the pressure cooker that was the intensive care ward. In order to visit Mark we had to pass through the larger intensive care ward which seemed to be crowded with babies and their families waiting for a donor. Mark had actually been quite far down a long wait list when he got his donation and it was heart wrenching to walk by the families who were still waiting, knowing full well that many of them (approximately 30%) might never get a donor. It was even worse for us knowing that we had jumped ahead of many of them; their eyes seemed to all turn and watch us as we walked through the ward. We had indeed been extremely lucky not only with Mark's A blood type but also his large birth size. Had he been even a bit smaller he would not have been able to use that donor's heart, and would have almost certainly died waiting for a transplant. All the other parents knew the circumstances and tried to be very supportive and happy for us but their joy was bittersweet because they knew that with every missed opportunity, the chances for their child were slipping away.

The preparations for leaving the hospital were not straightforward in spite of the fact that we only lived five minutes away. We had to take a basic first aid course and pass several tests. We had to read numerous manuals outlining routine care for a 'transplant infant' as well as emergency procedures. We were given a stethoscope and instructed on how to listen for an abnormal heart beat. We were to listen to Mark's heart at least three times a day and keep records of his heart rates. As the grand finale we had to do what was known as an overnight. A bed was set up for us behind a portable divider in Mark's area and we were responsible for Mark's care for the whole night. I felt like I was back at summer camp. The night was uneventful, so the next morning there was another meeting of the whole group of specialists prior to letting us out. Everything went along very nicely and numerous checklists were completed until it came to the part where they asked if we had any questions. I had only one simple question – Would I now be in charge of Mark's pacemaker and if so at what rate should his heart be beating? The cardiologists were on one side of the room and the pediatricians on the other side and we were sitting with Mark in the middle of the room; it was quite interesting. After much heated debate it was decided to remove the pacemaker and that was the end of that problem. All the cables, tubes, and wires were quickly removed – it was really quite frightening – how would we know that his heart was still beating?

How would we know that he was still alive?

Chapter 8
Counting the cost

For which of you, intending to build a tower, does not sit down first and count the cost, whether he has enough to finish it – lest, after he has laid the foundation, and is not able to finish it, all who see it begin to mock him, saying, "this man began to build and was not able to finish."

Jesus Christ, *the Bible*

A comparison between the Canadian and U.S. health care systems is one of the few things capable of stirring up feelings of national pride in Canadians. Many Canadians view health care in the U.S. as expensive and often inaccessible to average citizens. In Canada we often hear news reports of Canadians travelling in the U.S. and requiring medical treatments which result in very large bills. So when we were told we must travel to the California to seek medical treatment for Mark the first question I had was, how much would it cost?

The actual size of the estimated bill was indeed daunting but the range of error, if you will, amounted to tens of thousands of dollars. It was at first hard to imagine why a more accurate estimate was not possible but something as straightforward as the retrieval of the donor organ could result in a huge difference from one case to another. I had never considered the logistics of this part of the whole endeavour. I thought that the surgeons would be performing the transplant operation and at the crucial moment would ask for the donor organ and insert it. Someone involved with the donor would have removed the organ and would have sent it to them. This is not the case. The same team that performs the transplant operation actually travels to the hospital where the donor has died, assesses the suitability of the donor and the organs involved, harvests the organ they need, and travels back to do the surgery. Teams from Loma Linda have travelled as far as Montréal in Canada to pick up an organ. This involves a major undertaking: a chopper from the helipad at Loma Linda to a nearby Air Force base, a private jet to an airport near the hospital where the donor has died, and a helicopter ride to that hospital. The team then evaluates the donor organ and - if it is suitable - harvests it and packs it into a cooler filled with ice cold physiological saline. They then repeat their journey in reverse. At Loma Linda the sound of an incoming helicopter is almost certain news that another baby and their family will be getting the gift of life.

In our case we were very fortunate in that the little girl who died was local and the team could actually drive to the hospital. Given the congestion on the freeways in the LA area, it might have been tempting just to take a helicopter, but I am told they travelled in an ambulance to deal with the delays in traffic. The end result was that our bill for the retrieval of the donor heart was relatively insignificant compared to what it could have been. We were also very fortunate for other reasons. Mark waited in intensive care for only one week before they found a suitable donor whereas some babies wait for up to three months. He was only in hospital for two weeks after his operation – really quite a remarkable recovery time. Many babies were in intensive care for much longer post-op. Obviously, the cost for a day in intensive care can vary but even if one uses average values the difference between two weeks and three months results in huge savings. Mark has never been readmitted to hospital since his transplant, whereas many other patients needed to come back to spend time in intensive care to deal with complications, viral infections, or rejection episodes. A few even required a second transplant which would essentially double the cost.

Although we were very lucky in many ways our financial situation was more difficult for other reasons. Many families who came to Loma Linda had been living in their communities for years, often even generations. When the community heard of their situation local fund-raising organizations formed trust funds for the family and raised substantial support. As result some families had a large bank balance from which to draw emergency funds. This was not the case for us. Nicole and I had just moved to Saskatchewan from Ontario where we had been living within a transient student population. I did not know anyone in Saskatoon and we had no time to do PR work. The local Kinsmen Club did help us out with a small amount of money but we arrived in Loma Linda with student loans coming due, and credit cards and lines of credit at their maximum capacities.

Our recent move to Saskatchewan was the source of other problems as well. In Canada health insurance is a provincial matter. In order to qualify for Saskatchewan health benefits one must have lived in the province for at least three months. At the time of the diagnosis we had not met this requirement. As students you are covered by your home province regardless of where you live in Canada but we were no longer students and Nicole had not lived in British Columbia, her home, for at least two years and I had not lived in Manitoba for at least seven years. At the outset there was considerable confusion as to which health authority the physicians in Saskatchewan should submit their bills, and where they should seek approval for covering the costs of the transplant. It was finally decided that if Nicole left for California first and I stayed on in Saskatoon a bit longer I would maintain our address long enough to qualify and everything could be submitted to Saskatchewan Health.

There was only one small wrinkle in this plan which we thought might come back to haunt us: Nicole and I were not married. As we would be crossing international borders, and dealing with government agencies and health insurance plans, we decided we had best overcome our reservations about the whole marriage thing and get a license. The term 'shotgun wedding' took on a whole new meaning. Time was of the essence because Nicole had to leave. We decided that we should at least try for some semblance of the real thing and although neither of us was affiliated with any church, Nicole's grandmother had taken her to the Catholic Church when she was young so we thought we might start there. One afternoon we stopped in at the large Catholic Church in downtown Saskatoon and asked to speak to the priest in charge. We described our predicament to him as concisely as possible and he listened carefully for a while. He then began to question us as to our choice of the Catholic Church and our religious convictions. He asked us specifically if we prayed every day. We told him that due to recent events we would be open to consider almost anything, which was probably not the right answer. His response was that he could not marry us unless we attended his prenuptial classes which would be starting later in the fall. He then embarked on a long homily on how prayer was different from daydreaming. We had to cut him short and returned home where I got out the yellow pages and looked up the names of several Justices of the Peace in the phone book. We found one only a few blocks from our apartment and made an appointment for the next day.

The Justice of the Peace also wanted to interview us before he would actually proceed with a wedding. This interview went marginally better than the one with the priest. He agreed to perform the wedding ceremony on the weekend and told us his rates. He gave us a book of vows and asked us to choose which ones we liked. We didn't like any of them, mainly because they all contained some rather archaic language about husbands and wives; however with some serious editing on our part we finally came to a compromise on one of them. He was not happy about this but he was even more upset when he found out that we would not be having any rings at the ceremony. He thought that this was utter blasphemy but I insisted that going out and buying expensive jewellery was definitely not in our budget at this time. There was only the issue of witnesses left to discuss – we needed two people to sign for us and he suggested he could invite his neighbours at a cost of forty dollars. I made a quick phone call to one of my brothers who lived about two hours out of town and he and his wife agreed to drive in to officially witness the event and save us the forty dollars. So several days later the five of us stood in the JP's living room and we were married. The ceremony was lovely and particularly moving especially when we all looked down and noticed that the officiant was dressed very smartly in his best suit and tie but he was not wearing any shoes. We all happened to notice this at the same time and started to laugh. It was one of those situations where you try your best not to laugh but the harder you try, the funnier it gets. When he asked us what we were laughing about I told him were all just very happy. We have some lovely photos taken in his back garden; Nicole, very obviously pregnant, is holding a small bunch of flowers her parents had had delivered.

So now we had the paperwork in place and we could negotiate with the health insurance. At the time, coverage for an infant heart transplant was hit and miss. In the U.S. none of the major insurance companies would provide any funds, citing the fact that procedure was experimental. This continued to be the case until the mid-1990s. In Canada there had been only a couple of cases where approval was initially refused but after considerable pressure from the public, the insurance agencies in some provinces had reversed this decision and agreed to pay the in-hospital costs. Legally, if a patient requires care which can not be provided in Canada, the province is obliged to cover the costs of care outside the country; however the Canadian agencies did initially try to use the same argument the private companies in the U.S. had used to deny the requests. There appeared to be some variation from province to province but luckily for us there was a precedent in Saskatchewan – when we went down to Loma Linda there were already two other Saskatchewan families down there waiting for a donor for their babies.

In fact, a significant number of the first 100 babies who got heart transplants at Loma Linda were Canadian. This is true in spite of the fact that the population of the U.S.A. is tenfold greater than that of Canada. At first there was a suggestion that the incidence of hypoplastic left heart syndrome might be higher in Canada due to some environmental effects. You know – living in igloos and driving dog sleds may somehow be linked to having babies with defective hearts, or maybe it was due to the ink on our funny looking multi-coloured money? Studies later showed that proportionally the same number of American babies were affected as Canadian babies. This would suggest that either neonatal health care providers were not referring these babies, or families were choosing not to intervene for financial reasons. It raised the question – how often are people in the U.S. choosing not to seek medical treatment because they can't afford it? Living through this experience certainly made us extremely thankful for our public health care system in Canada. We learned of some heart-wrenching tragedies that American families had endured. In one case the family re-mortgaged their home and sold all their valuable possessions to come for treatment. Their child did not survive, and they were left with a large debt and no baby.

The large proportion of Canadian babies being treated at Loma Linda did not escape the attention of the media. At one point, several Canadian families were invited by a US media outlet to take part in filming a documentary about hypoplastic left heart syndrome. We were led to believe that the focus would be on raising public awareness of the desperate need for donors. When we arrived we noticed that only Canadian families were present. In fact the news team working in collaboration with a Canadian media outlet were trying to verify an idea that Loma Linda was aggressively marketing their program in Canada and grossly overcharging Canadian patients to subsidize patients from the U.S. As soon as we realized what was going on the whole show fell apart and I don't think anything ever came of it. I suggested if they wanted that kind of information they needed to check an audit of Loma Linda's financial records, not talk to us.

Before Nicole was admitted to the hospital for the delivery, I had only visited an American hospital twice. Both times were when we had been to the post-op transplant clinic at Loma Linda which was in a separate wing, so I had never seen the admissions side of things. At the post-op transplant clinic the staff was trained to work with parents of babies with major heart defects. They were definitely sympathetic to the fact that we were going through a traumatic experience. The staff members working in the general admissions department the night we arrived at the hospital with Nicole in labour were not at all empathetic. Their primary focus seemed to be on the financial aspect of the medical business. Having to produce a credit card prior to being admitted to a hospital was totally foreign to me. Also there was a bewildering array of signs on the wall indicating the type of health insurance cards that were or were not valid. How I wished that I was back in Canada where all you saw was a small sign politely asking you to have your government-issued health care card ready for the receptionist. I was used to a much kinder and gentler approach where, if in fact you forgot your card they could always, perhaps somewhat reluctantly and after a short and sweet lecture about not forgetting it next time, look it up in the system for you. I wanted to explain this to our somewhat belligerent gatekeeper that evening but it was very obvious I would be wasting my breath. Even after Americans have visited or have perhaps even been treated in a Canadian hospital they don't actually believe that we never directly pay any money to the doctor or to the hospital. This concept is completely foreign to them. They think there must be some catch. When they find out that it is actually illegal for the doctor or hospital to take remuneration directly from a Canadian patient they are convinced that all Canadians must be barking mad. As I handed over my credit card, I explained that if anyone attempted to charge anything to it the charges would be declined; it was in fact already completely maxed out.

Although I had heard much discussion about the Canadian public health care versus the private American system and thought I had understood the difference, actually I had a lot to learn. For the first two days that Mark was in the hospital everything was much too stressful for us to notice details related to costs and billing but as soon as we started to visit Mark in the intensive care unit on a regular basis that changed. Above his little bed, beside all the monitors, was a sheet with a lot of red stickers on it. We didn't really take much notice of it until one day Mark needed some ointment to treat his diaper rash and the nurse had some sent over. A small green tin of Bag Balm arrived with a red sticker on it. The nurse removed the sticker, stuck it to the sheet above the bed handed us the tin and said we should put some ointment on every time we changed his diaper. It was then that I figured out what all the red stickers were about; we had just bought a tin of Bag Balm, the same stuff I had used growing up on the farm to treat cuts on the teats of the milk cows' udders. Everything came with red stickers: packages of diapers, bags of IV fluid, catheters, etc. Periodically the sheet was taken down and the prices on the stickers were tallied up and billed to us. This was not something I had ever noticed in a Canadian hospital where most of that stuff is included in a daily fee per bed.

I had imagined that all the sheets of stickers as well as other bills were being sent to some central office somewhere and then a summary of all the costs was being forwarded to our health insurance in Canada which would then send a big cheque to cover the costs. It wasn't until several weeks after Mark's surgery when he was already out of the hospital that I realized things were not quite that simple. It was about this time that I started getting phone calls; sometimes from nice receptionists in various medical offices but also from some collection agencies. They were all looking for money to cover medical bills. I tried to assure them that the bills would be paid – our health plan in Saskatchewan would be covering everything. Most of the callers were ok with that with the exception of the collection agencies. They wanted the money *now*. A couple of them even sent collectors around to our front door. One particular young man was quite insistent that he get his money and told me that if I did not get him some cash by the following morning he was coming to repossess our car. I informed him that we had just purchased the car on one of those zero-down plans two months before and given the initial depreciation on a new car there was probably a whole lot more owing on the car than he would get for it if he tried to sell it on the used car market. He was not happy but he agreed to go away and let me try to figure out why he was not getting paid.

Because I kept getting calls and the callers were getting very persistent, I decided I had better look into the problem. I called our health insurance in Saskatchewan and it took several calls before I finally got to speak to the individual who was actually in charge of our account. He assured me that they were in fact paying our bills and when I gave him the information regarding the accounts which were outstanding, he told me that they had all been paid.

The problem was that one large cheque had been sent to cover all the bills, the idea being that there is some central office that would disperse the funds to the appropriate accounts. That is how I figured out that a central billing office did not exist. Each department, radiology, neonatal intensive care, the transplant clinic, as well as many of the individual physicians, had their own bill collection systems and offices. There was no coordination of billing and payment.

There was also another factor which contributed to the billing confusion in our case. When we were married, Nicole had not taken my name – said she did not want to be a Kroeker. She had been admitted to hospital under her family name and so our baby was referred to as 'the Robbins baby' for the first two days, which became Mark Robbins to some, while others were using the name on his birth certificate which was Mark Kroeker. Saskatchewan Health was paying the bills for Mark Kroeker. This problem was resolved after the first week but there were outstanding bills for Mark Robbins to be paid.

By talking to our man in Saskatchewan, I was able to establish which office actually had received the big cheque and when I called them, they assured me that, yes, they had received the money. In fact they were very friendly and happily informed me that we had a $30,000 credit with them. They knew nothing about any unpaid bills with other departments and when I asked them if they might apply our credit to the other accounts which were outstanding they told me that was not possible.

The next morning I paid a visit to the office that had all the money. I had taken to riding an old bike I had borrowed in an attempt save money on gas and my ride to the office turned out to be quite a wild adventure. I had expected the office would be associated with the hospital but it was actually in an industrial park in a rather dodgy area of a San Bernardino suburb. I spoke to the receptionist and explained our problem. Everything checked out, we did in fact have an excess of $30,000 in our account but using it to pay our other bills did not seem to be an option. I made several suggestions like transferring the money or having them write cheques to the other departments but nothing seemed to be possible. I was getting increasingly frustrated and at one point I was kind of thinking out loud and said that it was really quite ridiculous that they would have a large sum of money that did not belong to them. The fact that they had not informed anyone about this and seemed unwilling to give it up did not seem to be legal. What was I supposed to do – call a lawyer?

It was as if I had waved a magic wand at her – at the mention of a lawyer the receptionist immediately picked up her phone and within seconds a very nice man came walking down the hall and asked me to come into his office. I explained our problem to him and he confirmed that they could not write a cheque and give it to me and they could not transfer any money. He made a brief phone call, then turned to me and asked if I could wait half an hour. He could give me the money, but only in cash. Sure enough in about twenty minutes an armoured car showed up and two gun-toting guards came in with a large bag of bills and handed it to the receptionist, the cash was counted and signed for and then handed over to me. But what was I going to do now? I was on my bike in a dodgy area of San Bernardino with $30,000 in cash. Luckily I had my backpack with me so I stuffed the money into it and pedalled like crazy over to the hospital in Loma Linda, my heart pounding. There I got the addresses of the billing offices where we had accounts outstanding. I am sure everyone who saw me was wondering why I kept a death grip on my backpack the whole time. I then proceeded to deliver money. I paid the big bills first and I did not get quite finished by the end of the day, what with looking for addresses throughout the neighbourhood. That evening I suggested to Nicole we might go out for a fancy dinner and maybe some shopping - I still had a couple thousand dollars in my backpack. In fact we could pay off our student loans. We resisted the temptation, stayed home, and had beans for dinner again. The next day I paid off the rest of the bills.

So the health insurance was covering our in-hospital costs and that set of collection agencies went away, but other personal bills kept coming in and the banks started to insist we make payments on our student loans. The first few calls to the bank did nothing to convince them that perhaps in our situation we should be allowed to defer payments a little longer after graduation than was normally allowed. The managers in charge agreed that our situation was unusual but they still wanted their money. After more calls to the managers of managers, we did finally convince them to give us a break. But neither Nicole nor I was working and the other bills were rapidly piling up. We still had to pay rent, drive our car to the hospital for Mark's check-ups, and cover the extra expenses of caring for a special needs newborn. It was during this time that we discovered that even within Canada the health care system is not all the same. We became friends with a family from Alberta whose son also had a transplant and who were living 'in exile.' If you had Alberta health insurance all your costs were covered – their hotel room, meals, car rental, fuel, even their mortgage back in Alberta was being paid by the health insurance for as long as they needed to stay out of the country for treatment. It was like they were on an extended all-expense paid vacation. None of that was true if you had come from the rest of Canada.

When Mark was first born, while he was waiting for his transplant and then while he was in hospital after his transplant, we were very busy just being there for him. It was also an incredibly stressful time. Just managing his health care accounts was a full time job for a while; however, once things settled into a routine and Mark was home with us, I really needed to go to work to earn some money. Fortunately I was offered a job in a lab at Loma Linda University. Unfortunately before they could pay me I needed a work permit, a much sought-after commodity in California at that time. I needed to get this permit from the main immigration office in downtown Los Angeles. Some of the other Canadian families who had been at Loma Linda prior to us had managed to get work permits, however the process could often take up to 12 months. The coordinators in the transplant office had come to know a contact person at the immigration office who would apparently expedite a request for a work permit for families of 'transplant babies.' All I needed was the proper documentation from them explaining our reasons for having to stay in California.

I gathered up all the documents I was told I would need and headed for downtown LA. I thought I would try public transit; driving on the freeways could be a very frustrating experience during the day as traffic was so unpredictable. I found out where the bus for downtown stopped in Loma Linda – in fact it was on a lay-by just off the freeway. I missed the early morning bus because I did not realize that you actually had to flag it down. There were only three buses a day and the next one left at noon. I got on the noon bus which got me downtown at approximately three o'clock, but as soon as I found the immigration building I knew I was in trouble. There was a line-up of people extending from the front door for approximately two city blocks. I got into the line and after a few minutes tried to establish at what rate this line actually moved. This was difficult because almost everyone in the line was a migrant farm worker from Mexico and Spanish was the only language I could hear around me. I finally found someone much farther up the line who spoke some English and asked her how long she had been there. She told me two hours and when I indicated that I was at the back of the line she said I had no chance of getting in that day. I thought I had better at least try and I went and waited but sure enough just as I was approaching the front of the line, personnel from inside came out and announced they would be closing the doors in five minutes and we all had to go home.

The next day I was back on the freeway very early in the morning and this time I took my car. I arrived to line up at about eight o'clock in the morning but in spite of the fact that the building was not open until nine the line was already quite long. I think some of the people had spent the night. I did manage to get into the building this time and found that the purpose of the line outside was to sort people into lines on the inside of the building. I don't know what criteria were used for sorting, but I was in a very short line where we all spoke English while all the Spanish-speaking farm workers were in several long lines on the other side of the large entrance hall.

Ernest Kroeker

When I reached the clerk behind the desk, I showed him all my documents and he immediately informed me that the contact person known to the transplant coordinators no longer worked there. He suggested I make an appointment to see an adviser who would be able to help me. The first available appointment was two weeks later. I was starting to think I would never get a work permit but two weeks later I once again drove down and this time marched right into the building to my meeting. I was met by an elderly man who introduced himself as none other than the contact person Loma Linda had referred me to in the first place. What a surprise! When I told him that two weeks earlier I had been informed that he no longer worked here, he replied; "I retired but just last week agreed to return part-time to fill in for someone on sick leave." Unfortunately, now that he was no longer a supervisor he would not be able to expedite my application. He tried to make some calls to see if he could find someone who would do that but he was unsuccessful. His only suggestion was to submit all my paperwork and wait. He was not very hopeful that anything would happen for several months due to the large backlog of applications.

I was now convinced that the whole exercise would come to nothing and decided to have a cup of tea before I returned home empty-handed. The cafeteria in the building was very crowded so I was unable to find an empty table. I approached two men sitting at a table with empty spaces and asked if I could join them. I sat down and put my pile of documents down on the table beside me; on the very top was my Canadian passport. One of the men looked over and asked where I was from in Canada and what I was doing there? I told him my story and he listened with interest. Upon hearing of my futile attempts to get a permit, he said that if I could come up to his office right away he would help me. He was a special agent who dealt with foreign athletes playing professional sports in the USA and he worked with a lot of Canadian hockey players coming south to play for the NHL expansion teams. He said as long as I did not wish to stay in California for more than twelve months he could process my application immediately and give me a work permit. We went up to his office and within twenty minutes I was driving home with a work permit. I could start work the next day!

Chapter 9
Dr. Leonard Bailey

"Medicine is magical and magical is art.
The boy in the bubble and the baby with the baboon heart..."

Paul Simon, *The Boy in the Bubble*

In the fall of 1984 Dr. Leonard Bailey rocked the world when he transplanted a baboon heart into the chest of a baby girl. The world's media descended upon Loma Linda University Medical Center and a firestorm of debate and commentary was unleashed immediately. This operation caught and held the attention of millions of people around the planet as they watched and read about baby Fae's valiant struggle to survive, which ultimately ended with her death approximately three weeks after the operation. There was much controversy in the popular press and poets, philosophers, and pundits still discuss the ensuing story to this day. The verdict in the press was and still is definitely divided, one might even say polarized, around two positions. The man is either absolutely mad - driven to experiment with (some even used the word sacrifice) the life of a child in order to advance his own career as a surgeon and researcher - or he is a saint, boldly going where no one else dared to try and save the life of an infant who was born with hypoplastic left heart syndrome, which left untreated would surely have caused death shortly after birth.

The story was so controversial for a number of reasons. The use of a baboon heart raised huge red flags with a number of special interest groups and many in the scientific community. Animal rights activists were among the first to react and they were quickly joined by certain individuals involved with the sometimes bizarre but always entertaining evolution vs. creation debate in the U.S.A. Whole animals and animal tissues have been used in scientific and medical research for a long time, but to replace a human heart, which some less scientific among us even consider to be the seat of the human soul, with that of a baboon strikes at the very core of our being.

The animal rights activists were absolutely scathing in their attacks on Bailey. What gave him the right to sacrifice an infant baboon to try and save the life of baby Fae? I must say that I have never been clear about the notion of animals having rights. I have lived my whole life in close association with animals. I grew up on a farm with chickens, pigs, cattle, dogs, and horses and from a very young age was involved with the use of animals to produce food but I also have had some very good friends that were dogs and horses. I abhor the mistreatment and disrespect of animals so I can understand that animals have the right to humane treatment. What I do not understand is how people can invest so much time, energy, and money into animal rights when we still have children in many parts of the world suffering from malnutrition and diseases which could be easily prevented. We still have women disappearing from our streets downtown and it takes the police years to take any action towards finding the madman who took them home and slaughtered them.

In this particular case I can understand why killing an infant baboon for whatever reason would seem grotesque to many people, but when the motive is to attempt to save the life of a human infant I know what my position is. Given the choice between the life of a human especially a child and that of any animal I would have to side with the child. In fact I would have serious problems with someone who values the life of any animal above that of another human being.

Evolutionary biologists puzzled about the choice of a baboon rather than some other primate perhaps more closely related to humans, and this discussion brought to light one of the more interesting aspects of Dr. Bailey's persona. He is in fact a bit of an enigma in the scientific community as he definitely prefers the biblical account of creation to evolutionary biology and he is certainly not shy about expressing this view publicly. Shortly after Mark's surgery I attended a seminar on infant heart transplantation where Dr. Bailey spoke and in his talk he stated that the Creator had designed the infant heart and that this design made it easier for him to perform certain necessary procedures - not the kind of language one expects from a scientist and medical researcher. Needless to say, when the information that Bailey didn't believe evolution hit the popular and scientific press, criticism of him only intensified.

The eminent evolutionary biologist and natural historian Stephen Jay Gould used the baby Fae story in his monthly column in the *Journal of Natural History* to illustrate why scientists needed to clarify the confusion surrounding the use of the term 'homology.' Biochemists who often know little about evolutionary biology had coined the term 'DNA homology' which came to mean 'similar DNA sequences.' Evolutionary biologists had long before used homology to mean 'coming from a common ancestor' or as Gould states, "it is a quality of relationship based on evolutionary descent." Even though DNA sequences were similar they did not necessarily arise from a common ancestral sequence, so for quite some time there was considerable confusion as to what was meant by homology versus similarity. Gould was making the case that it was essential that the scientific community clarify this usage to avoid situations where scientists might "get it wrong" as he suggested Bailey did when he chose a baboon heart instead of one from a chimpanzee for example. Gould then goes on to say, "I just couldn't figure out how Bailey could work in such ignorance of known evolutionary relationships of homology – that is, until I read a chilling comment in the *London Times Higher Education Supplement*." Bailey's comment that Gould then quotes reads, "You see, I don't believe in evolution." Gould implies that Bailey's religious beliefs caused him to act in ignorance.

I have taught biology, cell biology, and genetics at the post-secondary level for almost 25 years and I would have to disagree with Gould. I would suggest if we were to venture out of our most ivy-covered of ivory towers we would find that the majority of medical practitioners, at least in North America, are shockingly ignorant of even the simplest basics regarding evolutionary biology. This would be true irrespective of whether they believe that the Earth and all life was created in seven days, or whether they believe that all primates evolved from a common ancestor, or whether they believe humans washed up on a beach in a clam shell aided by a raven. There is very little in medical education related to evolutionary biology. In fact, almost all aspiring young medical doctors I have met have very little interest in the subject and this is also true for those responsible for educating and training them. It is a situation which has always puzzled me. Most of the knowledge of biochemistry, molecular cell biology, and physiology upon which medicine and medical research are based comes from research on animal models. Yet when I suggest that it might be at the very least interesting to understand how the information from animal studies relates to humans the idea is met with indifference. It seems that it is more important that students of medicine can recite the names of all the bones and muscles in the human body on any given day of their final exam than to really come to a deeper understanding of the basic principles of biochemistry and biology.

It is interesting to note that the avid creationists who are also born-again Christians did not exactly rush to Bailey's defense but were for the most part silent on the issue. One can only speculate that they were unsure of what they should make of this situation or equally upset with the use of a baboon heart. For them, rebirth implies the cleansing and changing of the heart and soul (which according to some, sits on the heart) of the individual. How does one possibly reconcile the fact that the heart of a baboon - a non-human creature incapable of redemption - is now in a human?

As more people commented on and analyzed this story, the controversy only deepened. The rules and codes of conduct which are followed in any scientific research are very well defined and many researchers even consider them to be onerous especially as they relate to human medical research.

Major research grants are vetted at the institutional and national level by ethics committees and scientific experts in the various disciplines to ensure that no inappropriate research and clinical activity is going on. Experimentation with human and even animal subjects is very carefully reviewed and monitored before it is allowed to proceed. One definitely does not receive money or approval for research unless one reports this research in peer-reviewed journals or research seminars. The extreme view of some in the scientific community is that the granting of research monies and approval of research projects is too political and controlled much too rigorously.

Dr. Bailey did not meet the requirements to qualify for funding. He had taken a special interest in hypoplastic left heart syndrome during his training in paediatric cardiology. After sitting through yet another case review of an infant with this condition and listening to the team of experts come to the inevitable conclusion that the child would die, he challenged them to actually do something. When asked what he would suggest he stated that the child needed a new heart. His suggestion was always dismissed by his mentors and so he struck out on his own - on a mission to make his idea happen. He went along largely unnoticed, without any significant funding, doing research into xenograft heart transplants. He could not get major research grants and his research results were not widely published. When he spoke with colleagues about using baboon hearts in human infants they dismissed the idea as highly experimental and definitely advised against it. Yet he was persistent and eventually he went ahead with the landmark baby Fae operation. Although he did advise the appropriate administrative officials within his own institution before proceeding with the operation, he never sought the ethical and scientific approval of any of the medical or scientific community at large. One can only assume that had he done so he never would have been given approval. Because of this, many in the medical community view his actions as brash, unethical, and highly inappropriate - some even suggest criminal. Dr. Kenneth Stoller, in an article in the journal *Perspectives on Medical Research*, states that Bailey's actions were unethical and unlawful and that he should stand trial in a criminal court. He takes issue with the fact that Dr. Bailey discounted the Norwood procedure and that a human donor was never considered.

I certainly remember the controversy evolving in the scientific press as I was a young graduate student doing genetics research at the time. I was often drawn into discussions about this case with peers and mentors in the scientific community. I must say that at the time I was squarely on the side opposed to Dr. Bailey and the baby Fae operation and fell just short of condemning him as a career-crazed mad scientist. I was not really in any of the special interest camps at the time and the story did not relate to me on a personal level so I did not get very emotionally involved in any of the arguments. I certainly got the lasting impression, however, that Dr. Bailey and his story were a bit crazy – he was probably a brash, overly-aggressive American surgeon. My opinion was stereotypical of Americans in general and surgeons more specifically.

As soon as I heard that we would need to go to Loma Linda if we choose in favour of a transplant for Mark, memories of the baby Fae story came flooding back. It was with this image of Dr. Bailey that I arrived in Loma Linda five years later. I was quite anxious to meet him as he was legendary with the parents of children with hypoplastic heart syndrome. He was seen as the man who would be able to fix the problem.

In fact it was not until some time after Mark's transplant that I first saw Dr. Bailey during one of our clinic visits with Mark. He had been away from Loma Linda during the time we were waiting for a donor and for the actual operation. It was Dr. Gundry, a colleague who had recently joined the team at Loma Linda, who did Mark's transplant. I was not too happy about that. Did this understudy really know what he was doing? Why did we not get the Maestro himself? What did he think he was doing abandoning the ship just when we needed him?

I was pleasantly surprised to find that the mental image I had of this man was wrong in almost every way possible. He was anything but brash and aggressive - in fact he seemed somewhat shy and unassuming. The morning I first saw Dr. Bailey, the clinic was particularly busy with many families in for their post-op clinic visits. Often both parents as well as older siblings would accompany the patient to the clinic. It was immediately obvious that Dr. Bailey genuinely loved children. He definitely paid more attention to the children - the patients and their siblings - than to the adults who were present. When he spoke to the kids he would kneel right down so he was literally on their level and his face would light up with a smile. He could quietly calm both the most worried parents and the screaming children that even the best of nurses had given up on.

We would get to know Dr. Bailey quite well because when Mark was several months old he was chosen as the poster boy for a documentary news clip which CNN produced on infant heart transplantation. The filming took place over several days and although Dr. Bailey was not present for much of it, it was very interesting to watch him speak with the media. We got to see all the out-takes which are often more interesting than the film itself. He was very humble about his accomplishments and not at all defensive, even though he was asked some tough questions and was still obviously painfully aware of some of the negative press he had received over the baby Fae operation. One got the impression that he tried to be open, honest and straightforward in answering all the questions he was asked. This was certainly not the case on the other side of the conversation with the journalists asking the questions.

We had agreed to be involved with the project on the condition that it would be used to help raise awareness for infant cardiac donors and had been assured that this was one of the primary objectives. When the piece aired, however, it was a strange story with cardiac transplant and the Norwood procedure pitted against each other in some sort of weird competition over which was the best option. When I checked with the PR people at Loma Linda, they'd also had no idea that this was to be the nature of the project. They were equally perplexed that the focus was definitely not on promoting infant heart transplantation.

Chapter 10

The teleological suspension of the ethical

"On the other hand, Hegel is wrong in talking of faith, wrong in not protesting loudly and clearly against the fact that Abraham enjoys honor and glory as the father of faith, whereas he ought to be prosecuted and convicted of murder."

Kierkegaard, *Fear and Trembling*

There are many similarities between Abraham's binding of Isaac and Bailey's baby Fae operation. In both cases the life and death of a child rests in the hands of a man wielding a knife. Both Abraham and Dr. Bailey defined themselves with a single act of faith and established a great legacy. Abraham is considered the father of the Jewish, Muslim, and Christian religions. As such he helped establish the beliefs, civilization, and development of much of the world as we know it today. Dr. Bailey has gone on to international renown, a true pioneer in the field of cardiac transplant in infants. He has not only saved the lives of hundreds of babies born with hypoplastic left heart syndrome but also taught many other surgeons how to do the same.

Both men have been accused of having some difficulties with full and open disclosure. Abraham arose early on the day of his journey to the top of Mount Moriah and set off almost too quickly in response to the divine commandment to sacrifice Isaac. In *Fear and Trembling*, Kierkegaard suggests that this is admirable in that Abraham does not procrastinate and dither about, questioning himself, questioning God, and worrying about the details as any normal person might. Rather he starts out early, immediately obedient to God's command to sacrifice his son. Kierkegaard even has Abraham kissing Sarah good-bye that fateful morning. In my opinion this explains why Kierkegaard was having some problems with his dear Regina Olsen at the time he wrote Fear and Trembling. Although he did a bang-up job of understanding Abraham, in the case of his understanding of Sarah, not so much.

I do not agree with Kierkegaard's take on the motives for Abraham's quick departure that morning. There is of course a completely different explanation for his apparent haste. Can you imagine what might have transpired had he met his wife Sarah as he was leaving that morning with their son, the donkey, the servant and a pile of wood? One can be pretty sure she would not have approved of his intentions to sacrifice Isaac. How could he have explained his divinely-inspired plan? Maybe he was simply ensuring that Sarah was still asleep when he left, like a delinquent husband sneaking out of the house early on a Saturday morning to play some golf or do some fishing instead of going shopping for things for the house as planned the night before? What could Abraham have told Sarah, or even Isaac for that matter, about his journey and plans for Isaac at the top of Mount Moriah?

Many in the medical community also accuse Dr. Bailey of "leaving a little too early" with the baby Fae operation.

Most medical ethicists would argue that Dr. Bailey did not adequately consult with his peers and obtain appropriate approval for the operation. Immediately following the baby Fae operation and even in the late 80s Dr. Bailey was under intense pressure to put the infant heart transplant program on hold until there had been a broader discussion of ethical issues. There was widespread consensus that parental consent was not being handled properly and that Bailey was just offering the families of infants false hope. The long term prognosis for these babies was not clear. No one knew for certain that the transplanted hearts would grow with the children. Maybe Dr. Bailey was just creating a time bomb and the kids would never survive past childhood. The estimated life expectancy for adults was 12 years post-transplant.

But Dr. Bailey refused to stop. He had faith that what he was doing was right, not only for the babies and their families but also for society. Dr. Bailey was suspending the opinion held by the vast majority of medical practitioners and, honestly, if I had been sitting on a review board discussing this issue I would have decided in favour of the majority. But I was not on a review board, I was sitting in a small room desperately happy that at Loma Linda there was hope of saving the life of my son. Like Abraham, had Bailey conducted himself as his peers thought he ought to, he might never have embarked on his journey.

We can only speculate what Abraham told Sarah and Isaac about his intentions on Moriah or if he told them anything at all, but we do know that Dr. Bailey did seek the informed consent of the parents in the case of baby Fae. But what did Dr. Bailey discuss with baby Fae's mother before proceeding with the operation? What could he discuss?

In fact how meaningful is the consent of the mother of a child, a layperson with little scientific knowledge, under these circumstances? The child is certain to die without an intervention and the procedure is both very unpredictable and highly experimental. It really becomes the classic devil and deep-blue-sea decision on the part of the parents. Baby Fae's mom was convinced that Dr. Bailey was not the devil and in the deep blue sea there was at the very least a plan to look for a glimmer of hope. Fae's mother's decision to sign that consent form and Bailey's decision to proceed were in fact courageous acts of faith.

It is precisely the similarity between Abraham's and Bailey's dilemmas which is most intriguing. Both stories are perplexing and confusing when one is standing on the outside looking in. The dilemma in both cases presents us with a problem which Kierkegaard describes as the teleological suspension of universal ethics. It is interesting to note that he states that the ethical is suspended, not violated, broken or even ignored. With both Abraham and Dr. Bailey, their defining act is one which when viewed from a rational, disengaged perspective is highly unethical. I would certainly not want to be a judge or juror involved in the trial of either of these men. Yet the question is one which I believe all of us must deal with. Each of us at some point in our lives comes to the realization that our real purpose in life is to define ourselves – in fact maybe that is what life is all about. That is our life's work if you will. This is our own personal *anfechtung*. But the real dilemma is that self-definition is something we can never achieve by struggling along within the universal. It is only when we step out of the universal and examine the very core of our being that we can find purpose and meaning in our own lives and in the universe.

Our first response is often to conform to the universal. We believe that we can define ourselves by becoming members of the group. We chant the right mantras, we join the right clubs and organizations, we train for specific jobs and careers, we graduate from very special schools, we don't do drugs, we don't tell lies (at least not big ones), we stop at red lights even though it is two in the morning and there is no traffic. We are taught from a very early age that the most important thing we can do is fit in with the rest of society. In fact fitting in to the group might actually be an inherited instinctive behavior in humans. Our teenage years, that period of our lives when we are obsessed with figuring out who we are, are filled with angst and turmoil exactly because of this problem. Perhaps we have it all wrong?

In order to become a member of the human race we must, by an act of faith through infinite resignation, suspend the universal. We must turn our backs on the group in order to become an individual and it is precisely then and only then that we become completely human. We must reject the notion that the herd instinct defines us as humans and become selfishly individual in order to find meaning and fulfillment within the group. So the particular individual suspends the universal (ethical), and is no longer concerned with the limitations and requirements of the universal. In so doing he gives himself and the universal meaning. Rather than follow the ethics of his day, Dr. Bailey helped re-write the book on ethics. Rather than follow the moral code of his day, Abraham becomes the father of the Jewish, Muslim, and Christian religions.

Ironically, through an act of faith the individual transcends the universal and in so doing attains a true sense of community and belonging which can only exist after the suspension of the universal. In the same way, the divine transcends ethical morality (in today's terms perhaps 'political correctness' should be used here). Mere religious adherence to moral codes and ethics does not lead one to the deity. It is only by an act of faith that morality and ethics take on real meaning and we move from empty ritualistic religion to true spirituality. The irony is that this act of faith appears to violate the very community and religion to which we aspire.

There is one final aspect regarding the comparison between the baby Fae case and the binding of Isaac which is noteworthy. Kierkegaard goes to great lengths in order to distinguish between a tragic hero and the knight of faith. In this particular case, Dr. Bailey is more like a tragic hero and Abraham is as always the knight of faith. This is not to diminish Dr. Bailey's monumental work of faith. He was willing to put everything on the line in order to do what he believed to be the right thing — saving the lives of babies with hypoplastic left heart syndrome. He had little in the way of rational justification for his actions. When we first arrived at Loma Linda one of the first questions we asked was whether or not the transplanted heart would grow along with the baby — something one might expect should have been worked out before undertaking such a transplant. Cardiac transplantation was becoming almost routine in adult patients where a mature human heart was used as a donor organ but the infants had a long life ahead of them and it was hard for us to imagine that a foreign organ was going to develop perfectly along with them. But even to such basic and fundamental questions, Dr. Bailey and his team had no definitive scientific answers. It seemed that Dr. Bailey was quite literally flying on a wing and a prayer. Yet he was willing to risk not only his reputation but even his career as a surgeon on pioneering infant heart transplantation. He was willing to commit what even today many academics in the field of medical ethics consider a criminal act to do what he believed to be right.

In the case of Abraham, one could argue that he was greater than Dr. Bailey for a variety of reasons. He too had no rational explanation for his actions. He was risking his entire dream of becoming the father of a great nation and he was committing a most heinous crime by attempting to kill his own son. But the sheer magnitude of the crime or the risk is not important in the establishing the grounds for the distinction between the tragic hero and the knight of faith. We can now assess both these acts of faith with the advantage of hindsight. In Dr. Bailey's case we can see that in the end the infant heart transplant programs he pioneered, not only throughout the US but also globally, justify his actions. History vindicates Bailey. For Abraham there is no such historical justification possible. The majority of us still look upon the binding of Isaac with absolute horror and dread.

I wish to close this chapter in the manner with which I started it, with a quote from Kierkegaard. I should however warn the reader that the following quote contains a very long sentence and uses logic which on first (and perhaps even second and third) reading appears to be totally illogical. "Faith is precisely this paradox, that the individual as the particular is higher than the universal, is justified over against it, is not subordinate but superior — yet in such a way, be it observed, that it is the particular individual who, after he has been subordinated as the particular to the universal, now through the universal becomes the individual who as the particular is superior to the universal, for the fact that the individual as the particular stands in an absolute relation to the absolute. This position cannot be mediated, for all mediation comes about precisely by virtue of the universal; it is and remains to all eternity a paradox, inaccessible to thought."

My own personal journey to Moriah could not be characterized as either that of a tragic hero or a knight of faith. Perhaps "a scientist goes to Moriah" would be most fitting. When we first learned of Mark's condition I was filled with dreadful despair; I felt utterly alone and afraid. I was very worried that we would make the wrong decision and live to regret the consequences for the rest of our lives. I could not think of anything other than my own particular problem. I kept going over and over the problem in my mind and could not see a way forward. When I turned my eyes toward Moriah I had very few other options. I recognized that by responding to *anfechtung* through resignation I could suspend the universal. I realized that the ethical did not matter – the opinions and limitations imposed by the universal were not relevant. The problem was not like a puzzle I could understand. That realization resulted in a feeling of peace and rest. It was as if the sun broke through the clouds and the winds died away. I did not need to struggle to understand our dilemma or to do the right thing. I was conscious that I was very much alone and I could not explain to anyone how I felt or why I felt the way I did. In spite of the fact that I had suspended the universal, it was precisely when I did that that I suddenly felt an overwhelming sense of oneness with all of life – with all living things. In many ways our decision seemed to be contrary to the universal or ethical. If we had been faced with the same situation even ten years earlier there would have been no choice to make – Mark would have died shortly after birth. An intervention was certainly not what would happen in the natural world. Also I had serious problems justifying a huge investment of resources to save the life of my child when so many other children in the world were losing their lives as a result of very minor problems which were relatively easy to solve. Why was our situation in any way special compared to others? And yet I was choosing a chance of life over certain death.

By virtue of infinite resignation – the first movement of faith – my life is no longer a struggle to understand. I am also not haunted by the fear of having made the wrong decision and I can now live with a measure of rest and peace. Moving from resignation to faith I have also gained the assurance and – I hesitate to use the term in this context – the knowledge that no matter what the future brings for Mark, we will be ok.

Chapter 11
A Way to Know?

"I know that my Redeemer liveth."

Job, *the Bible*

In the home where I grew up pretty much everything was forbidden on religious grounds. In certain instances the forbidden activities were explicitly stated: the use of alcohol and tobacco, dancing of any kind, going to the movies, watching television, a long lingering look at someone of the opposite sex, even so much as the appearance of gambling — so dice and playing cards were out of the question. In other cases it was often not clearly stated but rather implied by example. Any aspect of popular culture was immediately suspect and the default position was that it was probably sinful. Reading for entertainment was not necessarily forbidden but certainly frivolous. It was clear that the only book that was really worth reading was the Bible. The only form of entertainment which existed was the "home entertainment centre" which was actually a piece of furniture. A large wooden cabinet on legs housed a turntable and stereo as well as a radio. The radio was seldom used — only in special cases to listen to an educational program on the CBC perhaps. However, we did have a small collection of LP records, large black discs of mostly religious music. Certain classical music with a strong religious influence was a favourite. In that particular genre Handel's *Messiah* was the music of choice – how could one go wrong? The libretto was taken almost entirely from the King James version of the Bible, the music harmonious and traditional with all the chords being resolved in a timely and Teutonic fashion; the fourth, the fifth, the minor fall and the major lift.

We had a recording of the highlights of a live performance of the Messiah on which the late, great Elisabeth Schwarzkopf was the soprano soloist. I clearly remember being absolutely enthralled by her rendition of the aria, "I know that my Redeemer liveth." It is truly one of those rare musical moments, the high soprano, the orchestration, a perfect match of text with tune, work like pure magic to send shivers down your spine. The message is also not lost in the medium for I remember thinking; "How does she *know* that her Redeemer lives?" How *can* she know that? I remember wishing that I might be able to make such an emphatic statement with respect to anything I might believe or know but I could not and I did not.

When I finished high school in the late sixties I vowed I would never go to university, much to the relief of my parents who had often expressed the opinion that it was the entrance gate to a broad road leading to corruption and death. However a short time later, influenced by the social mood of revolt and upheaval that was characteristic of the sixties, I aimlessly and unwittingly set off on a personal quest for knowledge and enlightenment. At first I dabbled in the arts, writing poetry and attempting to set it to music at times, but I had always done well at math and chemistry in school and I was quickly drawn into the seductive lore of the scientific method. I had no clear goal but I remember discussing the possibilities for a master equation to define the universe with my fellow students. I was completely caught up in a global academic shift which would see science displacing philosophy and theology to become the king on the campus.

It is probably difficult for most present-day students to imagine a time when science was not the tough kid on the academic block and that at one time philosophy and theology were the faculties most sought after. It is interesting to note that in the 1860s one of the most stellar examples of scientific discovery of all times was made in the garden of a monastery. Gregor Mendel did his work as a monk, not by choice but out of necessity. Mendel's work is often used today to illustrate just how science should be done. However until the early part of the last century all things scientific went largely unnoticed by society in general and most of academia. It was not until the 1950s and 60s that things began to change and some one came up with the idea that science was a way to know something. It is one of those ideas that seems so patently obvious that we don't really remember who first formulated it and when they did it. In fact it is an idea which not only changed academia as we know it, but also had a profound impact on society as a whole. This is due to the fact that the scientific method provides us with a most elegant and extremely powerful method of knowing something.

In the 1960s and 70s one small word in this idea was gradually replaced with another. Instead of thinking of science as *a* way to know something we started to view it as *the* way to know something. Academics and laypersons alike quickly recognized the power of the scientific method and public interest in science and funding for scientific research blossomed. Not only did the natural sciences flourish but it was also during this time that we saw the birth of the social sciences. Until then we had been content to study religion and politics, sociology and anthropology, human behaviour and economics, in the arts along with the classics, history, languages, music, fine art, and philosophy. During the 1970s and 80s it became increasingly difficult for disciplines in the arts to compete for funding with the burgeoning science disciplines. Not only that but if science was the way to know, what was the point of studying anything else? Although this was never actually stated quite that explicitly, the question was often implied. So sociologists became social scientists, students of political philosophy, political scientists, and so on. This idea began to permeate society as a whole. In the early 1900s if one wished to convince someone that he knew something to be true he would don clerical robes and perhaps put on a large and impressive looking bit of headgear and make a proclamation from a regal looking chair. A significant number of people on our planet were convinced that eating red meat on a Friday was taboo for the first half of the 20th century, until one day the pope reversed his decision and suddenly it was ok.

During the latter half of the 1900s the clerical robes were gradually replaced with the white lab coat, the headgear was no longer required but safety glasses were a nice touch. The regal thrones were replaced with lab benches and sophisticated looking technological gadgets. The general public had no clear idea what the gadgets actually were used for, or what the letters behind the names of the scientists actually stood for, or really what the scientific method was for that matter, but we all became caught up in the phenomenon. Because the scientific method is such an elegant and powerful way to know, it served society well and scientists made amazing contributions to the civilized world. Scientific progress however also had a negative influence on society – ironically it caused the modern world to become more and more detached from the realities of the natural world. It essentially crushed much of what might be considered traditional knowledge. Knowledge gained from experience passed on from generation to generation and intuitive knowledge were viewed as insignificant or even dangerous in most cases. We lost touch with the Inuit hunter who sets off on a journey at night in a blinding snowstorm without a map or compass and arrives safely at his destination, and other indigenous peoples who use knowledge gained from their elders to survive in the most hostile of environments. Intuitive knowledge in particular was viewed with considerable suspicion by the scientific community in spite of the great Einstein quote, "The only real valuable thing is intuition."

It is interesting to note that it is the mathematicians who are often the only academics who still discuss intuitive knowledge and any student of higher math knows how frustrating this can be. The math prof fills a whole chalk board full of equations and then states that if we see that this is all true then, intuitively the next chalk board full of equations is also true. Most students just hate when that happens. In fact the study of science has become more about learning the right answers than asking the right questions. Many students have told me they study science because at least there is a right answer, not like in the arts where it is up to the professor to decide how good your exam or essay might be.

It was during the late 1900s that the view that the scientific method was far superior to any other way to know began to shift back again. Due in no small part to the many women in academia, knowledge gained from human experience was again recognized as useful and important. Science and the way science was done also started to change dramatically just before the turn of the century. During the heady days of the 60s and 70s much scientific funding came from public sources, mostly government agencies. That changed in the 80s and 90s until today the majority of funding for scientific research is private. Large multinational drug companies give huge grants for medical research. Chemical companies fund research into the science of agriculture and forestry. Research into electronics and engineering is most often done in-house at major companies. Although there have been advantages to this type of private funding, it pushed scientific research down a slippery slope. Gone are the days when a scientist works as an unbiased, inquisitive mind, free to dwell on questions just for the fun of it. The emphasis is on getting useful results that can be published or, better still, patented. Results and information are no longer freely shared at scientific conferences but rather guarded as proprietary information. We are at considerable risk if as a society we continue unchecked down this slippery slope.

My own personal crisis of science came to a head the day I submitted my Master's thesis at McGill University. One was required to submit seven copies of the final draft of the thesis at a special office in an old historic building in the middle of campus. As is typical of most students, I had left it to the last day, due as much to procrastination as to reluctance. I travelled down to the office with several friends who were also in a major panic and when we arrived at the office with our boxes full of paper we stood in the long line with about 30 others waiting to hand in our work. As we shuffled our way forward in line I had what can only be described as a major panic attack. I left the line up and went outside with my box of seven copies under my arm and sat down on a park bench, sweating profusely. After some time one of my friends came out and sat down beside me and asked me if I was ok. We started to talk about my reluctance to submit my thesis. I told him that I did not want to hand mine in because I did not believe what I had written. When I pressed him, he agreed that he was in a similar position but he convinced me that this is normal and that I should just go ahead and do it. This experience led me to question the nature of knowledge and my belief in the scientific method. When I talked to other scientists I would often ask them if they believed their results. I got some interesting answers. Most of them admitted that they had serious reservations and wished they could afford to purchase or design a better instrument or method to measure certain parameters and generate their data. Over time I returned to my childhood desire to be able to really know and I came to an understanding that maybe the only thing we can know for sure is that we cannot know anything for sure.

It was one morning in September 1989 that I was obliged to seriously reconsider the way I could know something. Nicole's father had driven down to Loma Linda with her so that she would be on site for the inevitable heart transplant. We were anxious to get there and be ready and waiting. Flying down at a very late stage of pregnancy was not advised and I had to stay back to move our belongings out of our apartment and put various projects at work on hold. It was quite a difficult situation because we did not really know when or if we would return. If we found a donor and the transplant was successful we might need to stay in Loma Linda for up to a year, but we might well be returning much sooner if things did not work out. Nicole's father agreed to stay down in California until I was able to go down. He had been very supportive, finding a nice place for us to live and covering many of the costs of our move. When I arrived in Loma Linda he had to return to Vancouver for work; life goes on. To avoid the congestion on the California freeways, he left very early in the morning while we were still sleeping. He wrote us a note and left it on the kitchen table. The last line read, "I KNOW everything will work out." When Nicole read the note she was already upset. Her father had been the one last link to that sane world we had left behind, the last little bit of security in a future that was so uncertain and daunting. She reacted to the last line of the note, not as if it were a casual expression but as a statement of fact. "How can he possibly *know* that everything is going to be ok? Does he not understand how serious this is? Why would he say such a thing? Is he trying to patronize us?" It was in fact a very good question; How could he know?

To this day Nicole's father insists that he did not actually mean what he wrote, saying "It is just an expression one uses in casual conversation." The note however got me to think about conversations I had had regarding the binding of Isaac. Many dismiss Abraham's journey to Mount Moriah by saying that he knew he would get Isaac back again. In one short breath they march him up to the top of the mountain and triumphantly back down again with Isaac in his arms. They are in such great haste that one wonders why he even bothered to go. Why not just fire up the barbecue in the back yard? He could put some sausages on the grill and invite the Boy Scouts or some of Isaac's friends from the local youth group and they could all hold hands and sing *Kumbaya*. This view of the binding of Isaac trivializes Abraham's faith and we miss the notion that faith may in fact be a way to know. For me as a scientist the notion that faith is a way to know is controversial and even dangerous. What next? A research chair for astrology in the department of physics?

It was several months into our ordeal at Loma Linda that I came to an understanding that faith might indeed be a way to know. It did not come as a lightning bolt from the sky but gradually over time I too knew that everything would work out. You could argue that as soon as Mark was thriving with his new heart it was easy to come to this position. But this knowledge does little to minimize the agony and uncertainty which we even now sometimes feel about his future. It also does not mean that I am never scared sick about having made the wrong decision but in the times of serious crisis - when we thought he might be rejecting his new heart or when he was suffering from his first major viral infection this knowledge was a source of tangible comfort.

It was Einstein who said, "Science without religion is lame. Religion without science is blind." Fortunately, most of us have moved past the situation where scientific knowledge was used to discount all other ways to know. As a society we had become locked into some bizarre competition which often escalated into one of those us-and-them situations. Inevitably these situations always lead to a comparison of our best with their worst. Our planet is currently faced with some formidable problems and conflicts and it will take all of our knowledge to arrive at viable and sustainable solutions. Instinctive knowledge which many indigenous peoples still possess, intuitive knowledge of mothers and mystics, the experience passed on by our elders, along with the scientific method will all be necessary if we are to survive and prosper. Do not get me wrong - I am not suggesting we turn back the hands of time and declare open season for snake oil salesmen and witch doctors. I am instead suggesting that we move forward and respect and value all forms of knowledge, and that we should carefully consider faith as a way to know. I would certainly never abandon sound medical advice based on scientific principles when it comes to the ongoing care of Mark's condition. However in a strange, almost supernatural way I also know when we are doing the right thing. This sense of knowing is not something which I can explain or mediate to anyone else.

Chapter 12
Going Home

The road goes ever on and on
Down from the door where it began
Now far ahead the road is gone
And I must follow if I can.

JRR Tolkien, *The Hobbit*

Leaving the hospital's intensive care ward with Mark was the first step on our long journey home. It was like cutting the umbilical cord when the physicians removed all the tubes and wires from his little body. We still had to return to the outpatient clinic for regular nursing. Typically families would live in the Loma Linda area for a year so they could return to the clinic for regular visits, first on a day-to-day basis and then gradually on a weekly schedule. Similar to the period immediately post-transplant when parents would measure the progress of the baby using certain landmark events, parents would now measure progress by checking how often the physicians in charge wanted to see them. Regular clinic visits would involve a complete work up with chest x-rays, scans to image the heart, blood tests and a physical examination. The team of specialists in charge was really quite impressive. There were three or four transplant coordinators and one of them was always available for us to call or see if we had any concerns. A special team of paediatricians was in charge of following only heart transplant babies and one of them would do the physical exam during clinic visits. Someone from that group was also available 24/7. There were two fully qualified cardiac surgeons as part of the team: Dr. Leonard Bailey, who pioneered infant heart transplantation, and Dr. Gundry, who had just been recruited when the workload could no longer be managed by one surgeon. They were of course assisted by numerous fellows and residents in training. Several immunologists worked specifically with the transplant babies. Although the physicians and technicians working in the radiology and imaging departments were not dealing only with babies, we obviously required special equipment and expertise there as well. As one might imagine the support staff of specially trained nurses and technicians who often worked behind the scenes was extensive.

The 'mother ship,' as we came to call the hospital, was indeed impressive in terms of quality and quantity of caregivers. We grew to love her dearly but our relationship could not last forever. Weaning is always a struggle, perhaps more so for the infant than the mother, but it is also a major triumphant step forward in life. This is definitely how we felt about leaving Loma Linda. We were looking forward to going home with great anticipation, not only because it was a signal that Mark was progressing well, but also because we could finally get back to real life, including our careers and family, in Canada.

At the same time moving away from the incredible safety net provided by a world class medical team and the many friends we had made both within that team and with the other families in exile was both frightening and sad. We knew that we could always call and get advice and that we would be coming back for visits. This was very reassuring but it would not be the same as being right there. We decided we wanted to be as close as possible to Loma Linda so I had been applying for positions at universities in Alberta and British Columbia. We would go to stay with Nicole's parents near Vancouver until I found permanent employment somewhere in western Canada. Arrangements were made to transfer Mark's basic medical care to a group of physicians in Vancouver and we started planning our move home. Nicole flew back with Mark because a long journey in the car with an infant is never any fun. I drove the car packed with all our belongings. I bought a roof rack for the top and I think I must hold some sort of record for transporting the most stuff on and in a Dodge Omni. Everything worked out well until I got to the Canadian border and they asked me if I had purchased anything during my stay in the USA. We had been living in California for eight months and almost everything I had with me had been purchased there. I looked the customs official squarely in the eye and coolly gesturing to the whole car replied, "Yah, all this stuff." I was hoping he would be as excited as I was about unpacking and counting everything. Wrong. He was a lot more excited about it than I could have even imagined. We spent a lovely afternoon together unpacking everything and debating about the value of each item – he was most disappointed that I had no receipts.

Nicole also had an interesting time crossing the border to come home. She had taken her own travel documents as well as Mark's birth certificate. We had anticipated that there might be an issue taking a young child across the border without his father, so I had written a note with my consent. The problem we had not even considered was that

Mark was an American citizen, not Canadian. We had just assumed that because we were Canadians, he was also one of us. That is not how it works, so before Nicole could get on the plane for Canada she needed to do some paperwork. She had flown to Seattle first and was transferring to a flight for Vancouver. She did not have much time to make her connection so she was frantically running around the Seattle airport dealing with the problem. Fortunately there was a notary public at the airport who could authorize all the necessary forms. He worked in the basement, packing fish for export while he was not engaged with his more formal duties. Nicole managed to find him behind some shipping crates, swore several oaths at him and other appropriate officials, and he signed the forms allowing them to fly home.

We had not been in Canada very long when we realized just how good the team at Loma Linda was. We were obviously very impressed with this group while we were there but just like when comparing good red wines, the difference between exceptional and good only becomes very obvious when you try them side by side. The physicians we had been referred to in Vancouver were very good but they were not specifically trained for dealing with a heart transplant in an infant and many of them had only a passing interest in the whole story. They also were not coordinated into a group that worked together closely. This became very obvious the first time we needed to monitor the level of anti-rejection drug in Mark's blood. This had been done weekly at Loma Linda. While we were at the clinic for a check-up a nurse would take a sample and send it to the lab which would test to check if the drug level was within the appropriate range. In Canada we had to find a clinic that could draw the blood and then send it to a lab where someone actually knew how to do the analysis required. At Loma Linda if the drug level was a little off, the transplant coordinators would call us within six hours and tell us how to adjust Mark's twice daily dose. If we did not get a call we were to assume that everything was ok. By the time we arrived in Vancouver, we only needed to check drug levels once a month so on the appropriate day we began the process of finding the lab that could do the work. We went in and they took the sample one morning and we went home and waited for the result. After two days Nicole and I began to wonder if the fact that we had not heard anything meant that the levels were fine. We decided that perhaps we should call and confirm that the policy was the same in Vancouver and that no news meant everything was fine. I started to make calls and it took me about two days to track down the results from the sample. No one was actually responsible for checking on this information. The results had been sent to Mark's paediatrician, his cardiologist, and the immunologist responsible for following his case and they had filed the report in Mark's chart but thought that that was all they needed to do. When I finally spoke to them about the actual level they were not at all clear as to what the optimum level should be. I knew the levels we had used in Loma Linda but no one knew if the assay used in the Canadian lab was the same as the one in California. It took a few more phone calls to Loma Linda to check on this so that the coordinators in Loma Linda could advise the Canadian physicians as to how to adjust Mark's dose if needed.

It quickly became very clear to us that if something as simple as monitoring drug levels could fall through the cracks, the really big stuff might not be working as expected either. We consulted the heart transplant clinic for adults in

B.C. and discussed the issue with the team there. We had hoped that perhaps they could start to follow Mark's case. There were lots of adult heart transplant patients in British Columbia and a very good clinic had been set up for their post-operative care but because Mark was an infant we were obliged to stay with paediatric services – the adult clinic could not take Mark as a patient. As the director of the adult clinic pointed out, there were only approximately 50 infant heart transplant patients in the world at that time and although several of them lived in B.C., a special clinic for them was not cost effective. He suggested that we continue to rely on Loma Linda for advice and most of our care and that given enough time he would try to recruit the appropriate people on the paediatric side of the system. He did an amazing job because two years later Dr. Derrick Human, a paediatric cardiologist with expertise in transplants, agreed to come to the B.C. Children's Hospital. He has done a super job of taking care of Mark for most of his life and now that Mark is an adult we are very reluctant to have him transferred to the adult program. He trusts and respects Dr. Human, as we do, and we really do not want to leave that very special relationship.

We really have only ever had one major disagreement with the medical professionals with respect to Mark's care. It began in Loma Linda and continued on in Canada. The instructions we were given when we left the hospital regarding general hygiene dealing with a transplant patient were, in our opinion, much too restrictive and counterproductive. Some of the information was just common sense and good advice for parents of any newborn. There really is no need to expose the very young to a huge risk of infection at an early age. However other directives like carrying a spray bottle of alcohol disinfectant at all times and washing down everything our child might come in contact with or vacuuming our entire house once a day without Mark present, these we thought were misguided and excessive. The advice not to expose Mark to other children we also took with a grain of salt. He had just spent four weeks in a major neonatal intensive care unit full of infants, some were there because they were very sick. We went to the outpatient clinic, at first bi-weekly, where there were often up to ten other patients, some were there battling some very scary infections. So we should not let Mark play with the healthy neighbourhood kids in the sandbox? Certainly if we saw a child coughing and obviously suffering from an infection we did not take any chances, but we did not want to try to put Mark in a bubble. We had decided for the transplant because we wanted Mark to have a normal life. We understood that he was on drugs to suppress his immune system and that there were risks involved with that, but his immune system also needed to develop and function normally. It really is a fine balance in the transplant patient. You do not want the immune system to attack the donor organ, but you do need it to function normally in all other respects; mostly fighting off cancer and life-threatening infections. We felt that attempting to shield Mark from normal challenges to the immune system which would allow him to develop normally would be counterproductive.

At Loma Linda our decision not to play along with the rigid guidelines was treated with a sort of bemused indifference by the transplant team. I am not sure that they really believed all the hygiene instructions were necessary but they obviously needed to impress on the parents of the transplant infants that they could not take this matter lightly. Once they realized that we understood the important stuff they were willing to overlook some of the guidelines which might not be valid. The immunologist we were referred to in Vancouver was from quite a different school of thought. We only had the one meeting with him when we first moved. He definitely was keenly interested in Mark's health and wellbeing and was determined to give him the best care possible. He did a very careful examination of Mark and his medical history and then had a long interview with Nicole and me. Over the course of the interview it started to become clear to him that we were not following many of the guidelines and he was becoming increasingly agitated. Finally he said, "Ok, I can understand that you wish to let your child have as normal a life as possible but you wouldn't for example let this child play outside on the grass?" I decided it was time to end the interview and smiled and said, "Oh yes, he has definitely done that. We live on a small farm and keep some horses. The other day I was working in the barn and Mark was crawling around in the aisle (it had been freshly swept). I noticed that he was trying to eat a stray horse apple but don't worry, I didn't let him do it." I am just glad the man did not have a weak heart. Needless to say we were never invited back.

Chapter 13

What ever happened to Isaac?

May God bless and keep you always
May your wishes all come true...And may you stay forever young.

Bob Dylan, *Forever Young*

There are many unanswered questions about the binding of Isaac which are debated vigorously by members of all three Abrahamic congregations even today. Did Abraham actually kill Isaac? And if so how could he have gone on to become the father of the Jewish people? How old was Isaac at the time? Was Isaac really the son Abraham tried to kill? (Many Muslims believe it was Ishmael who was to be sacrificed.) What was Isaac's response to the incident on Moriah?

For me, one of the most intriguing questions is – how did this story ever get out? Some biblical scholars speculate that Sarah, Isaac's mother, found out about this incident and that the knowledge of it had a dramatic effect on her, perhaps even leading to her death. But there is nothing in the story to suggest Sarah was present on Moriah or that she had any prior knowledge of the event. In his portrayal of the binding of Isaac, Chagall has her looking on with an expression of great distress but she seems to be watching the whole thing from a distance. As far as I know, he is the only one of the artists who have documented this event who has depicted Sarah as having been involved in the story. Although it is an interesting feature (in fact it is because of this that his painting is a favourite of mine), there is no evidence to suggest that the situation, as he portrays it, is accurate. Sarah may have been responsible for broadcasting the story once she found out about it but it was probably not her who broke the story in the first place.

If we are looking for possible individuals who could have broken the story, there are of course the servants who assisted Abraham and Isaac at the outset of the journey. They were instructed to stay behind, a considerable distance below, while Abraham and Isaac went on up to Moriah. It is possible that they were curious about what was going down and followed at a safe distance without being noticed. Perhaps they observed the whole incident and reported back to Sarah. The problem with this explanation is that we know some interesting details which occurred at the scene of the binding of Isaac which would not really have been noticed from a distance. This would rule out the servants and we are really only left with the either Abraham or Isaac.

I would suggest that Abraham is the most unlikely of these two as I doubt whether he would ever have spoken much about what he went through on Moriah. It certainly is not something that would come up in casual conversation – "So how was your day"? "It didn't start out so well but in the end I did not have to kill my son, the object of all my aspirations." This is equally as unlikely at the dinner table at home with his family as it is in the coffeehouse surrounded by friends. A boastful admission on the part of Abraham is also unlikely - who could be proud of attempting to kill his own son? A confession is a definite possibility but to whom and why would he feel the need to confess?

Each time I try to piece together how this story might have originally seen the light of day I am left with only one prime suspect – Isaac. He seems to be the most likely candidate to have broken this story. It is easy to imagine that the events on Moriah had a profound effect on Isaac but it is also very likely that this story is not something Isaac would have wanted to discuss with many people. In fact it is difficult to identify with the post-Moriah Isaac character. He would have almost certainly suffered from what is now known as post-traumatic stress syndrome. He probably had some problems sleeping at night after Moriah, perhaps he even woke up in a cold sweat screaming bloody murder. Maybe his mother heard his cries one night and having already noticed a profound change in Isaac, got him to tell all.

One can easily imagine the family dynamic might have been somewhat strained after Moriah. Would Isaac have ever been able to trust his father again? In fact how could he really relate to a father like this? If Isaac respects Abraham for his actions after their return from Moriah, then Abraham becomes virtually God-like. Now Isaac would be trivialized by the sheer magnitude of his father's actions. Like us, Isaac feels that our/his own few and faltering steps in the general direction of Moriah are so insignificant that nothing we/he could do or say would really matter anymore.

If Isaac did not respect his father after Moriah then life would have become equally difficult. This family did not exactly live in a closely-knit neighbourhood – they had left their homeland many years before and were pilgrims in a sometimes hostile land. At this time it was common practice for parents to choose spouses for their offspring. We can easily see how his mother might have had some difficulties finding a young girl who was not only suitable but also whose parents would consent to their young daughter marrying him. He may very well have become known as 'that boy with psychological problems,' always acting out at school or social gatherings. And then there would be his father's reputation to live with – it is said that the sins of the father live on in the children. Would a tendency toward killing your own offspring "run in families?" Certainly a mother would get to know that her son had had a dramatic change in behaviour and she would get him to confide in her. So this would all fit with the idea that Sarah did not actually break the account of the events of Moriah but could have been responsible for publicizing the story.

We do know that once the story of Moriah became public knowledge, it only very gradually became the bedrock of the Jewish, Christian, and Muslim religions and culture and as such affects the lives of a large portion of the people living on planet Earth even today. However, it was not until long after the incident on Moriah that the binding of Isaac became a very important part of the Jewish faith. The fact that God eventually comes to be known as the God of Abraham in all three of the mono-theistic religions is due in large part to the events on Moriah. However Isaac does not play a central role in the development of any of the three "great" religions. It was only during times of oppression that the Jewish people began to take strength from and find meaning in the binding of Isaac but they never really gave Isaac a central role in the story. In fact it was only when Christians noticed the obvious parallels between the binding of Isaac and the crucifixion very early in the development of Christianity that Isaac really comes into focus. In the crucifixion story the focus is definitely on the Christ while in the binding story the focus definitely remains on Abraham. The sacrificial nature of Isaac which the Jews had always recognized but never really focused on would later become a much more important theme, especially during times of oppression.

The only part of Isaac's life other than the binding which is notable occurs when he is very old and incompetent. He was blessed with twin boys, the older was called Esau and the younger, Jacob. As the eldest, Esau should have inherited the family fortunes but Jacob disguised himself as Esau and tricked Isaac into making him the family heir, trading this birthright from his older brother Esau for a bowl of soup. Not a great contribution to humanity for Isaac. Perhaps Isaac suffered from the trauma of Moriah his whole life?

There are many ways that parents traumatize their children – just ask any teenager out on a family vacation with their parents. How many times a day is it possible for the parent to say or do something that absolutely mortifies their teenaged son or daughter? This too was one of my major fears when making my decision to proceed with medical intervention for Mark. Would this decision lead to something more traumatic than joyous in the long term? That fear persisted with me well into Mark's childhood. Quite early in Mark's life Nicole and I realized that many children who suffer from serious childhood illnesses are treated in an extraordinary fashion. This type of treatment often has a pronounced negative effect on the child's wellbeing and development. For this reason we always tried very hard not to let him be a "special" child. In spite of our best efforts Mark has always been very special. He has dealt with the

Ernest Kroeker

difficulties in his life caused by his medical problems with exemplary courage. He has lived his life to the fullest.

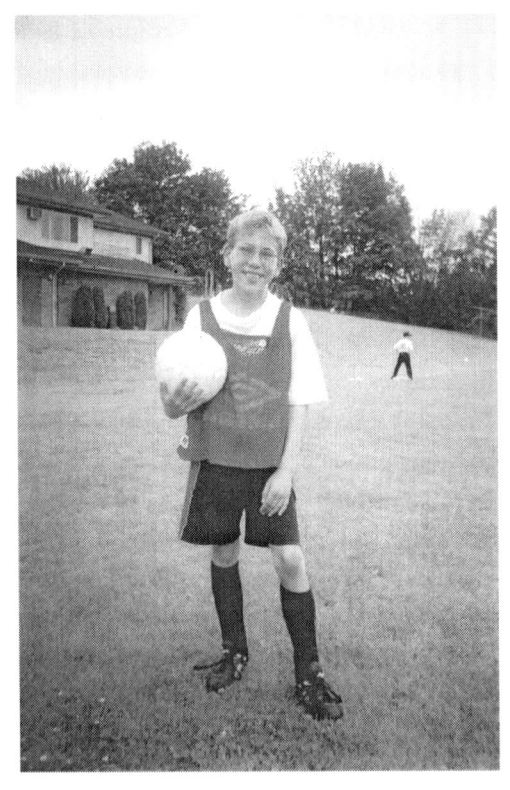

Always ready for a game of soccer

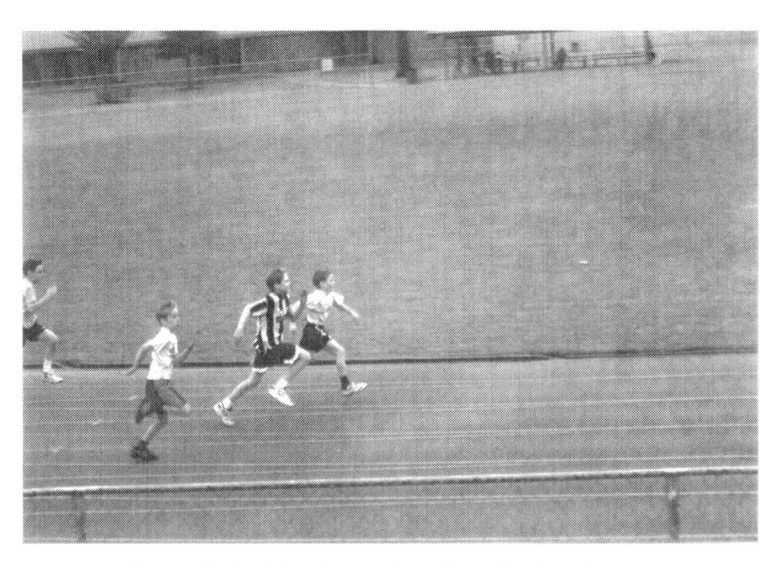

Mark (third) hitting his stride at the school track meet

As he was growing up we encouraged Mark to stay fit and active. In keeping with my own obsession, we drove him to weekly vaulting (gymnastics on horseback) practice and he won reserve champion at provincial level competition. He soon gave up riding horses because he preferred to play soccer and hockey, and watching him play has provided us with countless hours of enjoyment. Nicole's dad was also very helpful with Mark, taking him on marathon cross-country ski trips and bicycle tours.

Ernest Kroeker

Transplant recipient goes the distance

Mark Kroeker is a healthy, active, and enthusiastic nine year old who loves to go cross country skiing with his grandparents Sam and Janet Robbins. In the summer, when he is not out on the ski trails he plays soccer and basketball, takes care of his horse 'Tiki', is active in 4-H, and takes part in a special form of gymnastics done on the back of a horse.

Although he may not have won any first place medals, what makes Kroeker outstanding, is the simple fact that he is able to participate.

Kroeker was diagnosed at birth with a congenital heart defect and underwent a heart transplant when he was only seven days old.

Since then he has never looked back.

Kroeker, who lives in Deroche, BC, was in Salmon Arm this past weekend to ski in the Reino Keski-Salmi loppet held at Larch Hills. He accompanied his grandfather who was also at the loppet in an official capacity as Technical Advisor.

Kroeker only took up cross country skiing four years ago and has since managed to compete in at least one loppet each year. He says that he does not worry about competing, his times, or where he finishes.

"I just like being around all the people and being a part of everything that is going on. I do go as fast as I can though."

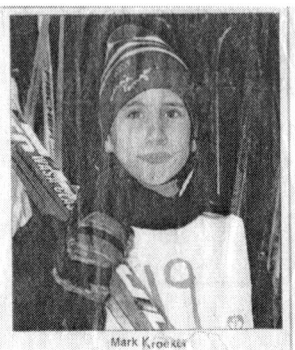

Mark Kroeker

reprinted with permission from The Salmon Arm Observer; Wed., Jan. 20, 1999 issue

Mark has always been the quintessential academic. He loved school and even as a child read everything he could get his hands on with a passion. Whenever we drove in the car he had to have something to read, so when I would forget to plan ahead I would stop at a service station and buy him a newspaper. He was not even in school yet when one day he informed me, very matter-of-factly, that the local newspaper really was not that interesting – in the future could I please buy him something like *the Globe and Mail*? He is keenly interested in his surroundings and absorbs knowledge like a sponge.

He has always been brutally honest - one of my fondest memories is the day I dropped him at school in second grade. We had had a disagreement that morning and I had lost my temper with him before we set off to school. We had driven to school in silence – he and his sister in the back seat, not venturing to speak. When he got out of the car I told him I loved him – he looked at me sternly, it was with the same intensity as that look when he was only five minutes old, and then he said, "There is no need to lie Dad."

Infinite Resignation

In first grade, he gave a brilliant performance in a dramatic production called "The Big Star," narrating the school Christmas pageant. He continued on in drama, when during his first year of high school he was invited to join the senior drama club and was granted special permission to do so even though he was a mere junior. He threw himself wholeheartedly into major roles, excelling not only as an actor but also as a director, stage manager, and in stage craft. He won awards for acting and stage production in high school.

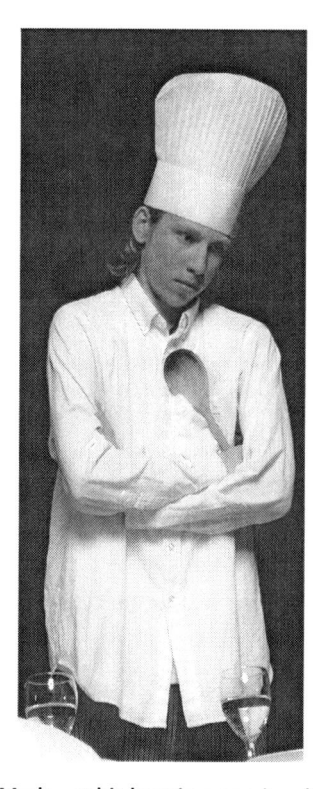

Mark – at his best in a comic role

He is currently completing a liberal arts degree at Mount Allison University where he is majoring in Geography

Ernest Kroeker

with minors in History and Philosophy. He is very active in student politics and has been re-elected as VP external for his student government.

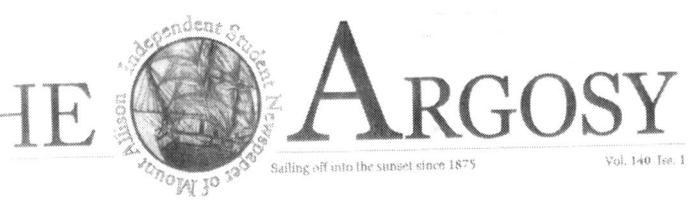

THE ARGOSY

Sailing off into the sunset since 1875 — Vol. 140 Iss. 1

exec members elected to NBSA exec

New Acting Dean of Social Sciences facing a hard year, with moxy

Sasha Van Katwyk
Argosy Staff

**Mark (left) at work in the Student's Society at Mount Allison University, reprinted with permission.
Photo credit - Lea Foy, The Argosy.**

I realize that pride is a vice and not a virtue, but I must admit that I have always been proud that he is my son. I can only hope that this transgression - my very public invasion of his private life - does not traumatize him too much.

Chapter 14
A horrible and somewhat lesser virtue

"Today nobody will stop with faith; they all go further. It would be perhaps rash to inquire where to, but it is surely a mark of urbanity and good breeding on my part to assume that in fact everyone does indeed have faith, otherwise it would be odd to talk of going further. In those old days it was different. For them faith was a task for a whole lifetime, not a skill thought to be acquired in either days or weeks. When the old campaigner approached the end, had fought the good fight, and kept his faith, his heart was still young enough not to have forgotten the fear and trembling that disciplined his youth and which, although the grown man mastered it, no man altogether outgrows – unless he somehow manages at the earliest possible opportunity to go further. Where these venerable figures arrived our own age begins, in order to go further."

Kierkegaard, *Fear and Trembling*

In the New Testament of the Bible it says that there are three great human virtues – faith, hope, and love, and that the greatest of these is love. There always has been and probably always will be much discussion about love and few would disagree that it is the greatest of human virtues. Humanity has produced great works of art celebrating, analyzing, eternalizing love. In North America there is a special day of the year set aside in honour of love thanks to St. Valentine and the Hallmark card company. Both these

Ernest Kroeker

venerable institutions have an equally nebulous history as protagonists of love.

Great philosophers and writers have established different categories to describe various types of love; the love of self - ego, brotherly (or sisterly) love - philia, parental love, romantic and erotic love - eros, love for our neighbours, the love of God. In fact many believe that God is love and that love is the only way to come to God. The great mystic and religious philosopher, Martin Buber, in his book *I and Thou*, wrote very eloquently and extensively about love and human relationships and how our relationships with others affect our relationship to God. The central teaching of Christianity involving love for your neighbour and the fact that "as you do to the least of those among you, you do unto me," never really made much sense to me until I read Buber. In his short story, *Martin the Cobbler*, Tolstoy beautifully illustrates this concept in terms of our real life explaining how love for your fellow human beings is in fact the way to find God. We all know the feeling of love and although it is abstract in that we cannot define or measure it, we can understand that it may be absolutely essential to the human existence.

Infinite Resignation

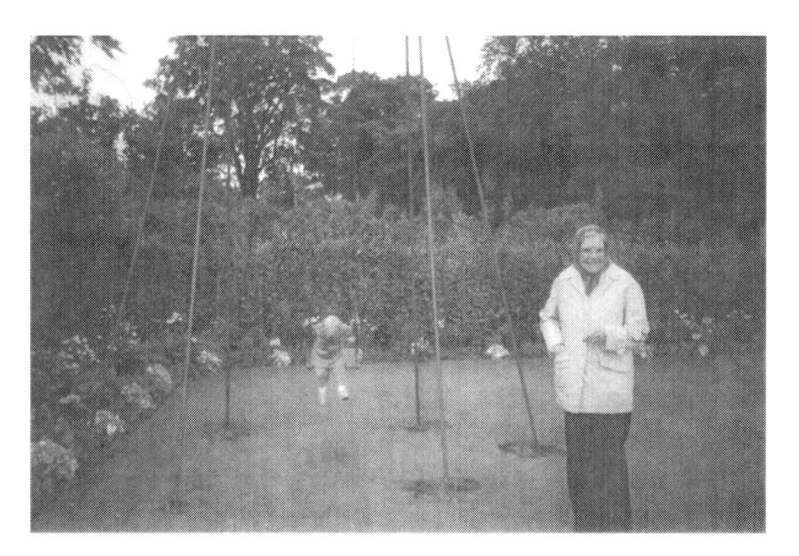

Mark's great-grandmother, Violet Robbins. She was known to her extended family as 'Saint Vi' because her whole life was devoted to loving her family, friends and neighbours. We travelled to Scotland so she could meet Mark as soon as he was old enough to make the journey.

Love is indeed the greatest of all human virtues and that would mean that faith and hope, the other two would be somewhat lesser virtues - or perhaps less virtuous? I would hope that everyone knows what hope feels like. Hope is also a virtue most of us possess and we understand that although it may not be absolutely essential to our existence, life is a whole lot better if we have hope. We can still hang on to life even though we have lost all hope but it really is not that much fun anymore. Hope is that stuff our dreams and aspirations are made of and what would life be without the ability to dream?

Faith, however is a virtue that we can apparently do without, for I have met even some very well-educated people who claim to have lost their faith, others claim never to have had it in the first place. They don't seem to miss it all that much. The idea that we can move beyond faith is not a new one. In *Fear and Trembling*, Kierkegaard goes to great lengths to try to convince us that this notion is pure folly. It has often been suggested in recent times that if we could put an end to faith the world would be a much better place. This suggestion has been made, due, in no small part, to the fact that people have observed that it is faith that motivates the suicide bomber. It has been pointed out that many wars have been fought in the name of faith and that although people also do good things in the name of faith, on balance faith is a horrible and destructive virtue, if indeed that is not some sort of oxymoron. I would not argue with the fact that faith is a horrible and potentially destructive virtue. We only need to consider the events on Mount Moriah to see just how horrible faith can be. It is this feature that makes faith very unique in the triad of great human virtues. While both love and hope, like faith, are not concrete, scientific concepts, and both can cause people to act in an absurd and even irrational fashion, they do not possess that element identified as the suspension of the universal or ethical. This combination of irrational behaviour and the suspension of the ethical is what makes faith a potentially horrific combination. People acting irrationally with no regard for reason is one thing, but add to that a disregard for ethics and the whole thing becomes not only lunacy but also lethal. It is little wonder that people single out faith as the culprit when identifying the central cause for acts of terror such as suicide bombings.

I too watched in absolute horror, along with masses of other people around the world, as the events of 9/11 unfolded and I certainly do not wish to minimize the grief and suffering of the thousands of families that were affected by that massacre. The event was particularly horrific because it was undoubtedly an act of terror motivated by religious fanaticism and the target was not military. But let us be honest, suicidal individuals eagerly volunteering for missions from which they knew they would not return have been around for as long as war itself. If they are on our side we call them courageous heroes who died for God and country (and may God bless those who are true courageous heroes) but if they happen to be on the other side they are heinous criminals and terrorists. The real irony of the situation is that the God they claim to be dying for is often the very same God on both sides. Dealing with the target of any type of attack can prove to be as complex as dealing with the motivation. There are rules of engagement, moral codes and international laws which exist to help us distinguish between war crimes and legitimate military action – and thank God for these. But it is here that we enter into a bit of a black box.

Some actions are obviously criminal and we can easily identify the person or persons responsible but if we take a careful look at the creative accounting and semantics involved with the casualties of war, things are often not that straightforward. The innocent civilian victims who suffer and die from starvation and the lack of proper medical treatment due to the destruction of a country's infrastructure during a war – would they be classified as collateral damage? The West supports, or even worse, sets up military dictatorships in developing countries to protect its interests in the region and then stands idly by and watches as these monsters and their people massacre tens of thousands of innocent civilian victims. How do we classify this - collateral damage? Or would this fall under the equally nebulous term of 'friendly fire?' And who is ultimately responsible for these deaths? Military commanders? Politicians or the people who voted for them? Counter intelligence agencies?

Considering for a moment that it was in fact possible, I am not sure that doing away with faith would actually mean that we would stop terrorism. Perhaps men like Ghandi and Einstein were correct when they suggested we should try a bit harder to do away with war itself. Although I am also no expert on the subject of suicide bombing, some people who are, have suggested that the problem is not that these people are motivated by faith but rather that they have no hope.

And how would one go about doing away with faith? Forcibly removing religious faith from people may have rather serious negative consequences. We can observe what happens by looking at our Indian reservations in North America. When the white man took the land from the aboriginals he also took the sacred connection these people had with the land and the flora and fauna it supported. When the white man also outlawed their religious practices the result was that he broke them. Even after several generations of attempted reconciliation it is not certain that they will ever live again. We can only hope that with enough love and prayer they will live again.

The notion that doing away with faith is possible and would help eliminate at least terrorism is based on a rather narrow definition of faith. For some reason faith has come to be defined as a set of religious beliefs - the word has become synonymous with religion. When we want to know to which religion one belongs we ask, "What is your faith?" But faith is so much more than merely a set of religious beliefs. Faith is multifaceted, just like love. We constantly demonstrate faith in our everyday lives; when we drive across a bridge we have faith that those who designed and built it knew what they were doing, when we travel on buses and trains or fly in aeroplanes we have faith in the technology and the operators of that technology, when we consume our food we have faith in those who produced and processed it. It might be possible to live our lives even though we do not have faith in others but it would indeed be a most primal state of existence. In the award-winning movie *Rain Man* Dustin Hoffman gives a brilliant portrayal of a savant, Raymond, who is pragmatic and analytical to a fault. Raymond refuses to fly on a plane or drive on a freeway and insists on buying his boxer shorts only at K-Mart. Without faith in others, if we must rely on only rational thought and reasoning to live our lives we are reduced to being phobic about almost everything.

We also must have faith in ourselves. This is often mistaken for a super form of self-confidence, sometimes even arrogance by people looking in from the outside. I am not a student of psychiatry, or even psychology for that matter, but I am told that there is a condition known as a catatonic state where an individual lacks the ability to move his or her body and in extreme cases does not speak. Maybe what is really wrong with these people is that they lack faith – even the faith that they are able to move their limbs and form words to communicate. Perhaps it is faith that provides us with the energy to live?

Faith has been very simply defined as the evidence of things unseen. In the physical world, energy has also been very simply defined as the ability to do work, as physicists often do. Although both these definitions can be useful, for me they are merely kind of cute and clever. There are some interesting parallels between faith and energy. Perhaps faith is to the spiritual world what energy is to the physical world. Both can be described yet not really defined. When we look upon them they can be both horrific and beautiful at the same time; a large wild fire burning out of control, a massive tidal wave, the perfect storm, Abraham's face on Mount Moriah. Maybe it is faith that provides us with the energy to live? It is faith that gives us the very energy to dream, perchance to love and, intuitively, you can see that if this is true then:

$$F = D^E$$

Where F denotes faith; D, the courage to dream, and as Einstein taught us $E = mc^2$.

One could further expand this formula and say that D is actually $A + R^\infty$, where A is *anfechtung* and R to the power of ∞ is infinite resignation.

(So there it is – that master equation I was searching for during those formative years at university. Ah, but "I was so much older then, I'm younger than that now.")

Imagine for a moment an absolutely idyllic scene. You are travelling in an open carriage through the peaceful countryside. Off in the distance on the hillside, a small group of singers and a string quartet are rehearsing Bach's Peasant Cantata for this evening's concert. The harmonious sounds wash over you. Below you, two lovers drift downstream in a rowboat on a stream where trout dart to and fro looking for unsuspecting flies. The lovers come ashore to find wild strawberries in a meadow where young sheep gambol, oblivious to the fact that soon they will be the special invited guests at dinner. A few fluffy white clouds in the clear blue sky do not obscure the warm sun on your face, softened by a breeze playfully blowing through your hair and carrying with it the fragrant scent of wild flowers growing along the roadside.

Let us stop for a moment to consider our mode of travel. The team of horses, sleek and muscular, trotting along in perfect step provide the energy for our journey, they represent faith. The driver, with almost imperceptible voice commands and slight of hand directs and guides our journey, the driver represents hope. The carriage, highly adorned and celebrated, of infinite value for it has carried princes and princesses to regal ceremonies, provides the vehicle which carries us to the divine; it represents love. All three of these components are vital to our journey. It is only when we possess all three of the great human virtues that our lives have meaning and we find peace and joy. Without hope, the team bolts off out of control resulting in a horrific wreck. Without love, we have no vehicle, we are nothing and we are going nowhere. Without faith, the horses, we have no energy and we are lame.

It is absolutely essential that we possess all three human virtues and that love remains front and center as the greatest of all virtues. Without love and hope, Mount Moriah becomes the scene of a brutal and horrific attempted murder where a father traumatizes his son beyond belief. Without faith it never happened at all. Although the great virtues share some common ground – they all defy definition and even reason, sometimes leading to irrational and even lunatic behaviour - there are some crucial differences. Love is extroverted, it takes us outside of ourselves. It can be demonstrated in a very public (universal) and obvious way between individuals. It can be mediated, we can easily observe it in the lives of others, we feel love for others, and in turn we feel the love of others. Faith however is a very private virtue which cannot be mediated - even the great father Abraham probably did not speak of it. It takes us out of the universal and into the very core of our being. Faith is a paradox which by its' very definition cannot be discussed.

When we demonstrate love to our fellow human beings we embark on a journey which takes us to infinity where we might see God. However, when we engage in Zen-like, infinite resignation we embark on a journey of faith to the center of our existence where we find out who we really are and where God might see us. It is faith which makes us unique and extraordinarily individual. It is love which can bring us together and make us infinitely human.

By virtue of infinite resignation we may live as if we were immortal even though we understand and know full well that we are mere mortals. Ironically it is when we suspend our own mortality and live as though we were immortal that we become completely human. Without faith we might sleep but we do not really rest. Without faith we might be satisfied but we cannot really find peace. It is only when - by virtue of infinite resignation - we stop acting instinctively and worrying about our basic human sensations and desires that we can start to truly enjoy a full life – rest and peace.

But faith and immortality and infinity are not destinations at which we can arrive. They are not possessions or goals we need to obtain or achieve. They are a state of mind - a way of being. As it is with infinity and immortality, there is no beginning or end to faith. We must keep going on with infinite resignation and it is then that we find peace and rest. However, all is not rest and peace at infinity. It is only in the eye of the storm, the center, where we find this incredible calm. The energy which is unleashed when we suspend our human mortality and live as if we were

Infinite Resignation

immortal is awesome – it can be absolutely horrific and it can be perfectly beautiful. When the suicide bomber walks into a crowded market square and commits a dreadful crime, he suspends his own mortality and acts as if he were immortal. The results are absolutely horrific. On the other hand Mother Theresa also suspended her own mortality when she spent her life loving the most desperate of individuals on the streets of Calcutta. The results were saintly. Dr. Bailey's life is more like Mother Theresa's because by faith he gave hope and life to many newborn infants with hypoplastic left heart syndrome. Father Abraham however might be considered the most dreadful of all terrorists. With one stroke of his dagger he could have wiped out all of Judaism and Christianity. But that is not how the binding of Isaac ends. In the end a divine intervention saves the day. It is love that wins the day for it is love, driven by the energy of faith which is guided by human dreams and hope, that is the greatest of all virtues. Faith however remains elusive – almost inaccessible – a horrible and somewhat lesser virtue.

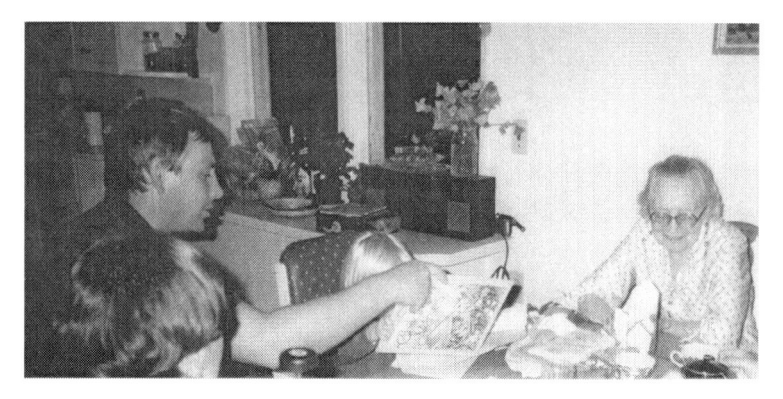

Mark's great-grandmother Helena Hamm. She traveled to Moriah and back several times. Her first husband went missing and was assumed dead in a horrific civil war. She and some of her children were then sent to a work camp in northern Siberia. She was an honoured guest at Mark's second birthday party.

Ernest Kroeker

Several years before Mark was born I had a conversation with a friend with whom I had gone to school. She was a young woman who had had a child very early in her life – many of her friends and family had thought much too early. I told her about my dreams and she asked me why I was so interested in having children. I told her I really loved children and I thought most children I met quite liked me. She looked at me rather sternly and told me that if I wanted to have children what I needed most of all was faith. At the time I dismissed this idea because I mistakenly thought that faith was that package of beliefs I had purchased wholesale at my local place of worship – many of which I had long since abandoned. After having my own children I realize that she was absolutely right. Having and raising children is the work of a lifetime which by virtue of infinite resignation might lead us to immortality.

Postscript

When I set out to write this book my primary objective was to increase awareness of and interest in organ donation. Organ transplants give life or improve the quality of life for thousands of people around the world. In North America, approximately 6000 people die each year because a donor organ is not available in time to do a transplant to save their lives. When asked, a large proportion of the general public say they support organ donation but only a small percent of these people actually agree to donate their organs. It is my hope that by sharing my story many people will consider becoming organ donors. There are many associations and societies with local chapters in most major centers that provide information and fund programs related to the promotion of organ donation and transplantation. I would urge everyone to contact one of these groups and do anything possible to help save lives.

This book developed into more than an autobiographical sharing of experience. As I was writing, it became a very personal account of how I came to a much deeper understanding of faith. I relied very heavily on the book *Fear and Trembling* to come to this understanding and this book formed the basis for many of the ideas in my own writing. I do not want to give the impression that I have some brilliant insight into faith or even Kierkegaardian philosophy for that matter. I still have many more questions than answers when it comes to the meaning of life. It is my hope that by honestly discussing my ideas I might inspire others to explore similar ideas in their own lives.

Another book from which I borrowed some ideas was *Abraham* by Bruce Feiler. This is a beautifully written book which inspired chapter 13. I wish to thank Mr. Feiler for writing a great book.

I have many friends and colleagues with whom I had numerous discussions about the contents of my book as I was writing. Without these interactions I would never have been able to write this book. I am sure that I will not be able to name everyone – so you know who you are – thank you all very, very much. I love you all.

This book is all about my family so to say that I could not have written it without them would be redundant. Nicole, Mark, and Robin, I hope that the next twenty-five years will be as interesting as the past twenty-five have been. You are the fulfilment of all my dreams – with the exception of that Grand Prix dressage test. I will always love you more than you can know.

CPSIA information can be obtained at www.ICGtesting.com
Printed in the USA
LVOW07s0601190215

427260LV00001B/21/P